CKD

STAGE 3 COOKBOOK

The Ultimate Guideline for managing Chronic Kidney Disease through Delicious and Easy-to-follow Low Sodium, Potassium, and Phosphorus Diet

TESSA E. MONROE

© 2024 by Tessa E. Monroe
All rights reserved.

No part of this book may be reproduced, stored in a retrieval system, or transmitted in any form or by any means—electronic, mechanical, photocopying, recording, or otherwise—without the prior written permission of the author.

This cookbook is intended to provide helpful and informative material on the subject matter covered. It is not meant to replace the advice and guidance of a professional healthcare provider. The recipes and information contained in this book are not intended as medical advice and should not be used as such. Readers should consult with a qualified healthcare provider for individual advice and recommendations.

The author and publisher disclaim any liability arising directly or indirectly from the use of this book. The reader is responsible for consulting a healthcare provider before making any significant changes to their diet or lifestyle.

First Edition: July 2024

TABLE OF CONTENTS

INTRODUCTION   7
1.1. Understanding Stage 3 Kidney Disease   7

BREAKFAST RECIPES   15
Apple and Cinnamon Oatmeal   16
Berry Oatmeal with Almond Milk   17
Scrambled Eggs with Bell Peppers and Mushrooms   18
Creamy Breakfast Polenta with Stewed Blackberries   19
Huevo Ranchero (CKD-Friendly Omelet)   21
Shakshuka   23
Pecan and Fruit Bowls   25
Green Pineapple Smoothie   26
Cottage Cheese with Pineapple and Papaya   27
High-Fiber Cereal with Berries   28
Baked Sweet Potato with Chia Seeds   29
Pear and Ricotta Toast   31
Low-Sodium Breakfast Burrito   32
Protein-Free Pancakes   34
Poached Pears with Ginger   36

LUNCH RECIPES   37
Vegetable Masala   38
Gumbo Z'Herbes   40
Thai Pineapple Salad with Carrot Cashew Dressing   42
Lemon-Herb Vinaigrette   44
Pumpkin Soup with "Chorizo" Mushrooms and Corn   45
Curry-Ginger Vinaigrette   47
Beet Salad with Candied   48
Smoky Corn and Chile Soup with CKD-Friendly Collard Greens   50
Tostada Salad   52

Smoky Collard Greens	53
DINNER RECIPES	**55**
Mexican Street Corn Salad (Esquites)	56
Veggie Fajitas	58
Portobello Steaks with Mashed Cauliflower and Balsamic Arugula	60
Italian Pesto Zucchini Noodles	62
Pineapple and Veggie Kebabs	64
Refreshing Vinegar Slaw	66
Louisiana Remoulade	68
No-Sodium Uwami Sauce	70
Summery Pepper Salad	72
Main Dish Salad	74
Ginger-Garlic Ramen Bowls	77
Tortilla-less Soup	79
Smoky Caesar with Charred Romaine	81
Jackfruit "Carnitas" Tacos	83
Watermelon Gazpacho	85
Mushroom Bourguignon	87
One-Pan Lemon Garlic Chicken with Veggies	89
SANCK OPTIONS	**91**
Curd and Crunch Cottage Cheese	93
Carrot and Creamy Hummus	94
Sweet Yogurt Parfait	95
Veggie Straw	96
Creamy Cottage Cheese & Berry	97
Rice Cake	98
Air-Popped Popcorn	99
Mini Veggie Skewers	100
Edamame Energy	101
Almonds and Apple	102

Berry Blast Smoothie	103
Feta and Dill Cucumber Refreshers	104

MAIN COURSES — 105

MEAT AND FISH — 106

Garlic Herb Roasted Chicken	106
Skillet Steak with Chimichurri	108
Stuffed Pork Chops with Spinach and Feta	110
Ground Turkey Meatloaf with Zucchini Noodles	112
Beef and Broccoli Stir-Fry	114
Cod with Tomato Caper Sauce	116
Shrimp Scampi with Zucchini Noodles	118
Tuna Salad with Celery and Avocado	120
Blackened Tilapia with Cajun Seasoning	122
Baked Salmon with Lemon Dill Sauce	123

SOUPS AND SALADS — 125

Chicken and Vegetable Soup	125
Creamy Keto Cauliflower Soup	127
Taco Soup with Ground Beef	129
Italian Wedding Soup with Meatballs	131
Lentil Soup (moderate portion)	133
Steak Salad with Blue Cheese and Arugula	135
Grilled Chicken Caesar Salad	137
Cobb Salad with Grilled Chicken and Avocado	139
Salmon Salad with Berries and Walnuts	141
BLT Salad with Turkey Bacon	143

DESSERT — 145

Fresh Fruit with Vanilla Syrup	146
Macadamia Nut Fudge	147
Creamy Keto Smoothie	149
Watermelon-Blueberry Sorbet	151

Raspberry Fool	152
Spiced Keto Cheesecake Bites	153
Chocolate Avocado Pudding	155
Lemon Ricotta Fluff with Berries	156
Sugar-Free Chia Seed Pudding	157
MEAL PLANS AND SHOPPING GUIDES	**159**
Grocery Shopping List	163
Tips And Strategies For Using The Grocery List And Lifestyle Changes For A Kidney Disease Diet	165
Using the Grocery List	165
Lifestyle Changes	166
APPENDICES	**168**
Appendix A: Nutritional Information of Common Ingredients	168
Appendix B: Conversion Charts	173
CONCLUSION	**177**

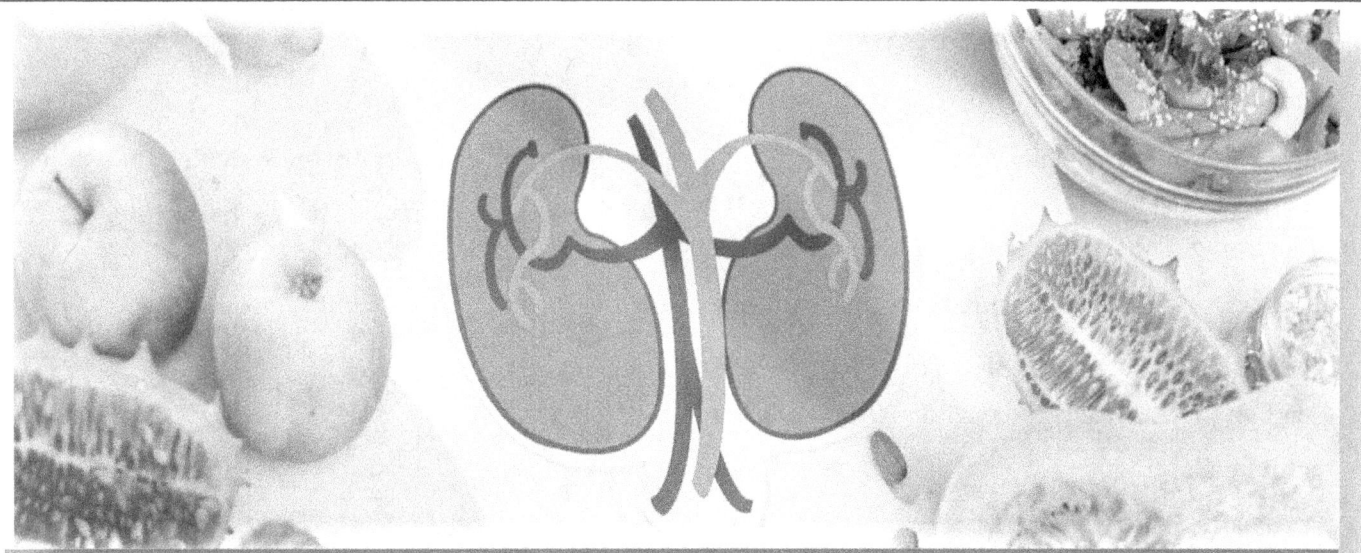

INTRODUCTION

1.1. Understanding Stage 3 Kidney Disease

You wake up in the morning. Have your breakfast, go to work, come back, spend time with friends and family, and finally hit the sack. The time in between these activities is spent without thinking twice about what it is - a gift. A body that is working perfectly without us even realizing its existence. To be aware of ourselves, our sense organs, our qualities is rare till when we go out and start our day. An active, hardworking and healthy being has the power to do all these things without the intervention of external medication. One of the powerful organs in our body that helps us to get up, go to work, and stand up to our expectations is the kidneys.

Stage 3 kidney disease marks a pivotal point in the progression of chronic kidney disease (CKD), characterized by a moderate decline in renal function.

This stage is clinically significant as patients begin to experience tangible symptoms due to the reduced glomerular filtration rate (GFR), which measures how well the kidneys filter blood. It ranges between 30-59 ml/min. The subdivision into stages 3A (GFR 45-59) and 3B (GFR 30-44) helps in tailoring patient management more precisely.

At this juncture, the kidneys are less efficient in filtering waste products and excess fluids from the blood, leading to noticeable health implications. Patients may encounter issues such as fluid retention, resulting in swelling, particularly in the lower extremities. The accumulation of metabolic wastes can cause systemic toxicity, affecting various body systems. Moreover, there's an increased risk of developing complications like anemia, cardiovascular diseases, and early bone disorders due to imbalances in minerals and hormones that healthy kidneys typically regulate.

Electrolyte imbalances, such as high potassium or phosphorus levels, alongside acid-base disturbances, become more prevalent, potentially leading to further health concerns. It's crucial for individuals at this stage to receive appropriate medical attention and lifestyle guidance to slow disease progression and mitigate symptoms.

1.2. Common Causes Of CKD

Diabetes is the leading cause of CKD in the United States, accounting for about 44% of diagnoses of kidney failure. High blood pressure is the second leading cause. Other conditions that damage the kidneys and cause CKD include, but are not limited to: glomerulonephritis, inflammation from immune response; interstitial nephritis, inflammation of kidney tubules; polycystic kidney disease and other kidney malformation; prolonged urinary tract obstruction due to disorders such as an enlarged prostate, kidney stones, and some cancers; prolonged exposure to toxins, heavy metals, solvents, or cigarette smoke; use of certain medications, such as certain antibiotics like gentamicin and vancomycin; and certain over-the-counter pain medications or allergy medications.

In addition to identifying the underlying medical condition which caused damage to the kidneys, physicians will also identify the amount of remaining kidney function the patient has by performing blood and urine tests. These tests will also allow for a determination of the rate of progression for the disease. Due to the progressive nature of CKD, early intervention is key to maintaining kidney function. For most, kidney damage is permanent and cannot be reversed.

1.3 Symptoms And Diagnosis

Symptoms of stage 3 chronic kidney disease (CKD) can be subtle but may include fatigue, fluid retention leading to swelling in the extremities, sleep disturbances, changes in urination patterns, and back pain. As kidney function declines, patients may also experience a decrease in appetite, muscle cramps, and high blood pressure.

Diagnosis of stage 3 CKD involves a combination of blood tests to measure creatinine levels and calculate the glomerular filtration rate (GFR), which indicates how well the kidneys are filtering waste from the blood. A GFR of 30-59 ml/min is indicative of stage 3 CKD. Urine tests are also used to detect protein or blood in the urine, which can signal kidney damage. Imaging tests like ultrasounds or CT scans may be employed to assess the kidneys' structure and rule out other conditions. A kidney biopsy might be performed in certain cases to determine the specific type of kidney disease and the extent of damage.

1.4 Kidney Disease Risk Factors

While most people value their kidneys, they rarely think about risk factors for kidney disease. The common kidney disease risk factors usually are linked to demographic factors. Demographic factors are age, gender, race, and ethnicity. Behavioral risk factors are those risk factors where an individual has the ability to modify or change their behavior. Behavioral kidney disease risk factors include obesity, sodium intake, cigarette smoking, hyperlipidemia, and physical inactivity. Environmental kidney disease risk factors include residence, lower socioeconomic status, and low levels of educational attainment. Chronic kidney disease may lead to faster heart disease and kidney failure.

It's important to understand the risk factors of Chronic Kidney Disease (CKD) so they can caution and screen those patients who are at highest risk for the disease. In doing so, healthcare providers should use a method that evaluates all individuals with any of these characteristics. It is time to think about this disease daily and begin preventative and treatment on those who are at risk.

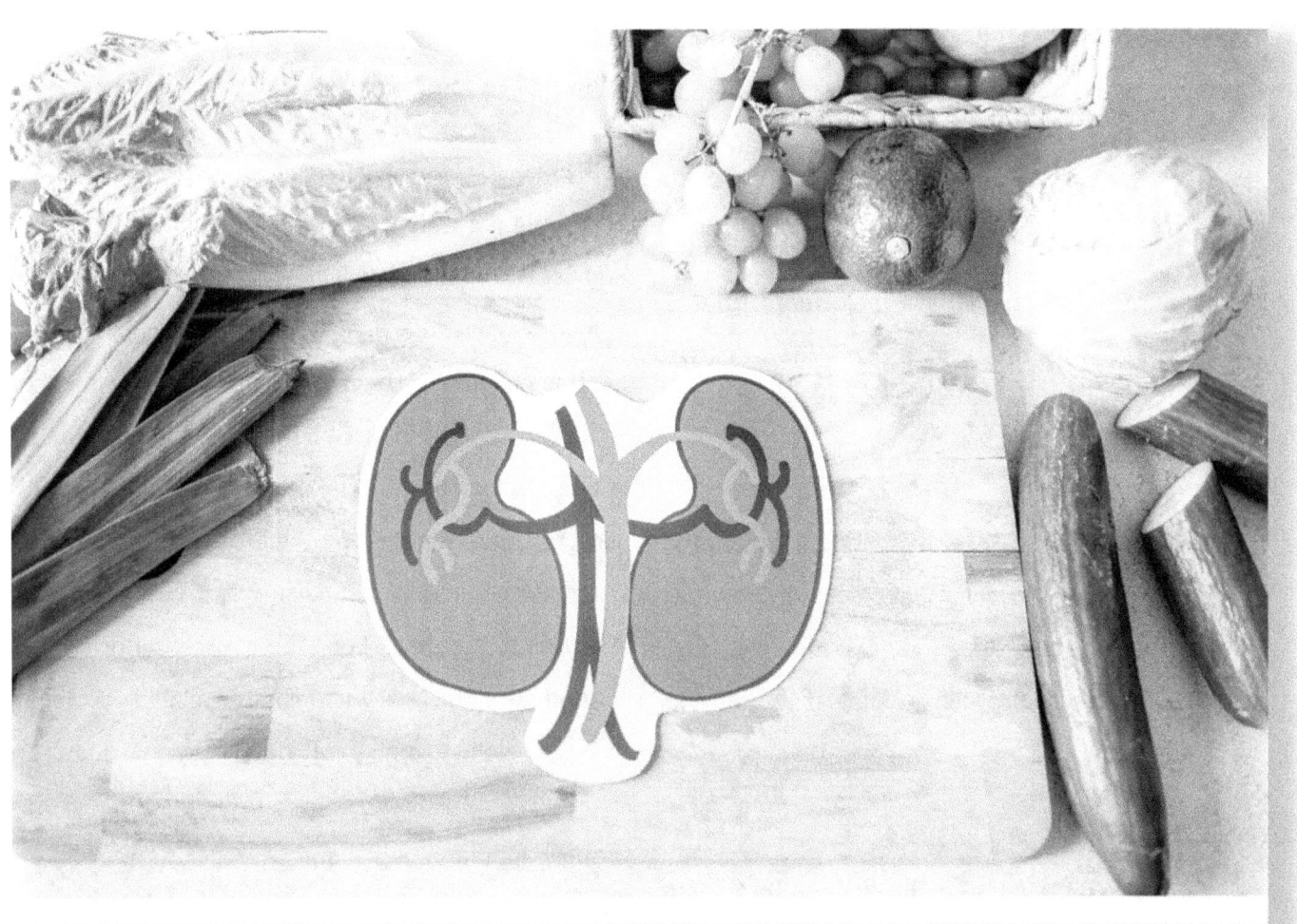

2. Nutritional Guidelines for Stage 3 Kidney Disease

People with stage 3 chronic kidney disease, also referred to as only stage 3 kidney disease, are at risk for developing progressive kidney failure. Their kidneys are not doing a good job of removing the wastes from the body. This can result in waste products building up in the blood and urine, which can lead to protein-energy wasting, bone and mineral disorders, sudden weight loss, and spikes in potassium and phosphate levels. The Sphinx strategy is followed, preventing further kidney damage by controlling high blood pressure and diabetes and avoiding medications that can damage the kidneys. Blood pressure and blood sugar control and medications that protect the kidneys will decelerate the process. The majority of stage 3 kidney disease is still coming from a healthy, low-protein, low-potassium diet. Our kidneys have more trouble processing waste products as the disease progresses. Individuals with CKD should consult with their

Your kidneys serve several important functions. The two most important ones are filtering out waste products from the blood and making urine. They also help control the amount of fluid in the body, make red blood cells, and help produce vitamin D.

Chronic kidney disease (CKD) is a condition in which the kidneys are not working as well as they should. Causes of CKD include diabetes, high blood pressure, low blood flow to the kidneys, and inflammation of the kidneys. Foods high in protein, potassium, and phosphate can cause the kidneys to work harder, so they should be limited. Others like dairy products, bread, and pasta can be eaten as the kidneys still work well. This book has over 80+ low-protein and low-potassium recipes. A plant-based diet with low-protein grains, breads, fruits, and vegetables is preferred

2.1. Importance of Diet in Managing Kidney Disease

By eating the right foods and having a listening ear and love for our body, whether it is your own or someone you take care of, it can be turned into healing. Patients with chronic kidney disease (CKD) are supported by the fact that their diets should face appropriately altered nutritional prescriptions based on their only available parameters that may influence diet if within normal American society. For the vast majority of individuals, these decisions are related to their average dietary intake of fluid, energy, sodium, potassium, phosphorus, and protein, changes in clinical parameters, their degree of nutritional status, in comparison to their existing medical care plan, and the specific nutritional goals that the provider struggles to fulfill in the nutritional care plan. Patients must be followed up closely due to the constantly changing nature of their renal disease. These guidelines would need to be reassessed on an ongoing basis.

A good diet is essential in your journey to a sound mind in a sound body. It is a well-known secret used for preventing or treating a range of ailments, but for kidney disease, there are extra benefits. To guide you, I have created this cookbook. This Stage 3 Kidney Disease Diet Cookbook is derived from the necessity of having realistic recipes to maintain good nutrition for those with Stage 3 kidney disease. With proper preparation and foods that work for you, the author can help maintain your quality of life with a good diet. The recipes here are designed to reduce the workload of the kidneys while providing a healthy diet.

2.2. Key Nutrients to Monitor

It is generally not a good idea to put a CKD patient on a diet high in protein when their kidney function is decreasing. People with CKD are often told to moderate their protein intake and are sometimes even told to go on a low-protein diet. However, as the CKD Foundation notes, the American Medical Association has stated the benefits of using cooking strategies and food consumption to manage CKD in lieu of taking pharmaceutical agents. Eating right can provide CKD patients with essential nutrients needed for bodily function and life. But, it is important for CKD patients to moderate certain nutrients, while maintaining other nutrients. The nutrients we must monitor in CKD patients, especially stage 3 CKD patients, are sodium, potassium, phosphate, calcium, protein, and some other nutrients such as lysine, arginine, taurine, etc.

Sodium: CKD patients need to monitor their sodium intake strictly to avoid high blood pressure, worsening of CKD, and fluid retention. High blood pressure and extra fluid can lead to heart attack, stroke, edema, pulmonary edema, heart failure, and further damage of glomeruli. Highly processed foods (frozen, canned, fast, most convenient foods), foods high in sodium (fast food, snack chips, pretzels, large pieces of corn chips, salt crackers, etc.), high-sodium seasoning, high-sodium sweeteners, table salt, and most salty foods (dips, soy sauce, etc.) should be avoided. A stage 3 CKD patient should have no more than one set salt (600 mg sodium) plus natural sodium from vegetables and fruits (low-salt vegetables, fruits, and tomato are encouraged) per day - or 650 to 1500 mg sodium, according to the recommended low-sodium diet.

Potassium: high blood potassium levels (hyperkalemia) are dangerous, even life-threatening.

On the other hand, low blood potassium levels are also dangerous for CKD patients. Healthy people should consume enough foods high in potassium because potassium is essential for bodily function. The recommended daily intake of potassium for healthy people is 4700 mg (4700 mg for males and 4700 mg for females). CKD patients, however, should not consume too much potassium when their kidney function is compromised. The reason is that their kidneys do not work like they used to. The excretion of potassium is mainly dependent on their kidney function and sometimes the potassium intake. It is very important to consume moderate levels of potassium to maintain normal blood potassium levels. The recommended daily intake (recommended daily allowance, RDA) by the American government is 2000 mg potassium per day. Because of the build-up of potassium, it can cause dangerous hyperkalemia. High-potassium is defined as a potassium content of over 200 mg per serving, a low-potassium content is defined as less than 200 mg potassium per serving, and a very low-potassium level is defined as less than 100 mg potassium per serving.

Overview of Nutritional Requirements

In Stage 3 kidney disease, it is important to monitor and adjust the intake of certain nutrients to prevent further kidney damage and manage symptoms effectively.

Protein: Why Monitor? Excess protein can burden the kidneys and lead to waste buildup in the blood.

- **Guidelines:** Limit protein intake to recommended levels, typically 0.6 to 0.8 grams per kilogram of body weight per day.

Sodium: Why Monitor? High sodium intake can lead to increased blood pressure and fluid retention, worsening kidney function.

- **Guidelines:** Limit sodium intake to less than 2,300 mg per day, with a goal of 1,500 mg per day for better control.

Potassium: Why Monitor? Impaired kidneys can struggle to balance potassium levels, leading to hyperkalemia, which affects heart function.

- **Guidelines:** Monitor potassium intake based on blood test results, typically aiming for 2,000 to 3,000 mg per day.

Phosphorus: Why Monitor? High phosphorus levels can cause bone and heart problems as the kidneys fail to filter out excess phosphorus.

Guidelines: Limit phosphorus intake to 800 to 1,000 mg per day, avoiding high-phosphorus foods like dairy, nuts, and certain meats.

Hydration and Fluid Intake: Maintaining proper hydration is essential, but fluid intake should be balanced to avoid overloading the kidneys. The amount of fluid a person should drink depends on

Their individual condition and medical advice. Generally, aim to drink enough fluids to stay hydrated without causing swelling or increased blood pressure.

3. Meal Planning and Preparation

Meal planning is key to maintaining a nutritious diet. Make sure that you incorporate fresh fruits and vegetables in order to receive the most nutrition. The following are some helpful tips for proper planning.

Meal Planning Guide: Get started with meal planning that will help you save time and money. Start with dinner - often time dinner serves as lunch the day after. Plan for the day, often there is no time for a sit-down dinner. You may need to opt for fast and easy foods.

Make a shopping list, knowing what you need will help you get through the grocery in record time. Plan and prepare meals that will help you enrich your health. Eating at home does not have to be a dead-end chore. You can prepare healthy and delicious meals quickly and easily. Prevent eating the same meals over and over again. Give new recipes a chance, enjoy meals that stimulate your sense of taste.

Batch cook and have extras of each of your favorite meals. In instances of busy days, there is no time. Go easy and have a convenient meal. Keep easy-to-poach fish fillets - all you do is drop this satisfying food in for a quick and tasty meal.

Improve your cooking skills by learning some quick and easy meal ideas. Eating well gives your body the strength and energy that it needs in order to improve and heal itself. Eating the right types of food at the right time will also help you make sure that you are not gaining weight while your activity levels are slowing down. Eating the right foods will help with the healing process. Be sure to include a variety of fruits and vegetables, whole grains, and lean proteins in your meals, as well as a variety of different nutrients. Eating healthy foods can help prevent other types of diseases and complications from kidney disease, such as high blood pressure, diabetes, and heart disease. A healthy diet will not only improve your life but will also, more importantly, help you to live.

Preparing a shopping list is highly recommended so that you may purchase all necessary items for the meals that you will be preparing. This will save you time and money for other things. Keep a well-stocked pantry for convenience. Cook fresh foods in bulk whenever possible.

Then store in individual serving containers what you do not use right away in order to have meals on hand for the rest of the week.

Choose recipes that require only a minimal amount of preparation time. Use kitchen appliances that will save time - items such as a blender, slow cooker, and a food processor can save a great deal of time.

3.1. Balancing Protein, Sodium, and Phosphorus

As for mineral concerns, with reduced kidney functions, removing waste becomes more difficult. If the kidneys were left to process more waste, phosphate would build up and weaken bones. Unlike normal kidney functions retarding phosphate build up, there is potential for an earlier stage 3 to move to a later stage 3 during the loading. Decreased protein means phosphorus levels can be reduced as well. Since most phosphorus comes from animal proteins, you may still have more phosphorus building up.

There are vegetarian proteins that are high in protein, such as lentils. Lowering sodium intake is always the goal.

Products that state "sodium-free" or "salt-free" have less than 5 mg of sodium. "Low sodium" with the label will contain 140 mg of sodium or less. Each individual will have preferences for specific nutrient intakes by products, reversely the serving size can be reduced if your intention is to balance the food intake.

If your phosphorus is high, you may need to limit portion size if your meals contain high phosphorus levels.

For stage 3 chronic kidney disease (CKD), some of the concern shifts towards the remaining life of the kidneys. There is no longer a push to provide your kidneys with more protein. Instead, finding a balance between not enough and enough protein is key. Although you're advised to limit salt and sodium intake, without too much protein, it can make your meal less appetizing. This book will provide variety and savory foods to assist your kidney functions with the required nutrients. Whether you have high or low potassium levels, there are choices for everyone. Your renal dietitians will be pleased to see that you are enjoying these meals without the fear of additional nutrient intakes.

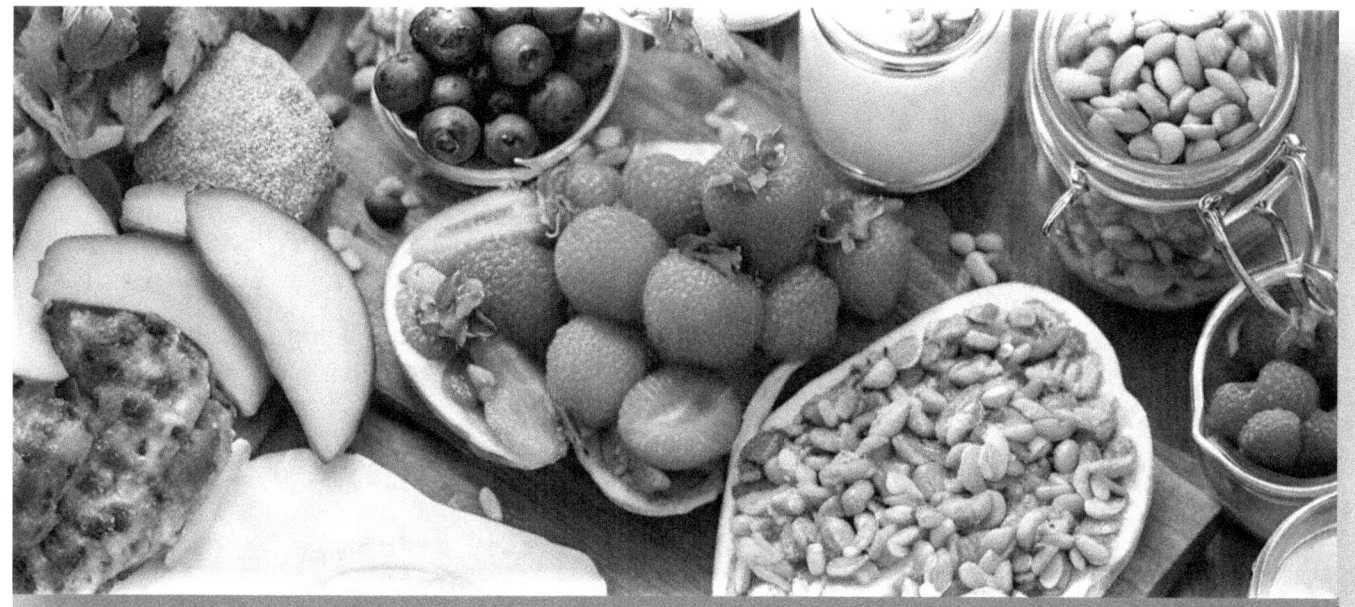

BREAKFAST RECIPES

Breakfast is often called the most important meal of the day, and this holds especially true for individuals managing Stage 3 kidney disease. A nutritious, balanced breakfast can provide the energy needed to start your day while adhering to the dietary restrictions essential for kidney health. In this section, you will find a variety of breakfast recipes specifically designed to be low in protein, potassium, sodium, and phosphorus. These recipes are crafted to not only support your health but also to delight your taste buds.

Each recipe includes detailed ingredients and step-by-step instructions, making them easy to follow. From hearty options like Berry Oatmeal with Almond Milk to refreshing choices like a Fruit Salad with Coconut Flakes, there is something for everyone. By incorporating these recipes into your daily routine, you can ensure you're starting your day with meals that support your kidney functions.

To make the most of these recipes, consider the following tips:

1. **Preparation:** Plan and prepare your breakfast ingredients the night before to save time in the morning.
2. **Portion Control:** Stick to the recommended serving sizes to avoid overconsumption of key nutrients.
3. **Substitutions:** Feel free to substitute ingredients based on your taste preferences and nutritional needs, ensuring they remain kidney-friendly.
4. **Consistency:** Regularly incorporating these recipes can help stabilize your nutrient intake, supporting overall kidney health.

By following these guidelines and enjoying the diverse range of recipes provided, you can make breakfast a delicious and kidney-friendly start to your day.

Apple and Cinnamon Oatmeal

Warm your mornings with this comforting CKD-friendly oatmeal. Apples add a touch of sweetness, while cinnamon provides a fragrant twist. This recipe is low in protein, potassium, and phosphorus, making it a great choice for Stage 3 CKD patients.

PREP TIME: 5 MINUTES | COOK TIME: 15 MINUTES | YIELDS: 1 SERVING

INGREDIENTS:

- ½ cup rolled oats
- 1 cup water
- 1 small apple, diced
- ½ teaspoon ground cinnamon
- 1 tablespoon chopped walnuts (optional)

COOKING INSTRUCTIONS:

1. In a saucepan, combine rolled oats, water, and cinnamon. Bring to a boil over medium heat.
2. Reduce heat to low and simmer for 15 minutes, or until oats are cooked through and creamy, stirring occasionally.
3. Stir in diced apples and cook for an additional 2-3 minutes, or until apples are softened.
4. Remove from heat and top with chopped walnuts (optional) and enjoy!

NUTRITIONAL INFORMATION: (APPROXIMATE VALUES PER SERVING)

Calories: 180

Phosphorus: 60mg

Protein: 3 grams

Sodium: 10mg

Potassium: 70mg (depending on apple variety)

TIPS FOR MODIFICATION:

- For lower potassium: Choose apple varieties lower in potassium like Granny Smith apples.
- Protein adjustment: If needing to further limit protein, skip the walnuts or use a very small amount. You can add a sprinkle of ground flaxseed for a slight protein boost and added fiber.

Berry Oatmeal with Almond Milk

This quick and easy oatmeal recipe is perfect for a heart-healthy and delicious CKD-friendly breakfast. Packed with fiber and antioxidants from berries, it keeps you satisfied without straining your kidneys.

PREP TIME: 5 MINUTES | COOK TIME: 15 MINUTES | YIELDS: 1 SERVING

INGREDIENTS:

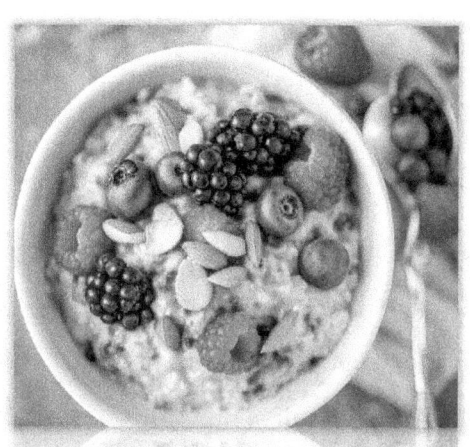

- ½ cup rolled oats
- 1 cup unsweetened almond milk
- ½ cup frozen mixed berries (or fresh berries in season)
- ¼ teaspoon ground cinnamon
- 1 tablespoon chopped walnuts (optional)

COOKING INSTRUCTIONS:

1. In a saucepan, combine rolled oats, almond milk, and cinnamon. Bring to a boil over medium heat.
2. Reduce heat to low and simmer for 15 minutes, or until oats are cooked through and creamy, stirring occasionally.
3. Remove from heat and stir in frozen berries. Let sit for a few minutes to allow berries to thaw slightly and soften the oatmeal.
4. Top with chopped walnuts (optional) and enjoy!

NUTRITIONAL INFORMATION: (APPROXIMATE VALUES PER SERVING)

Calories: 200　　　　　　　　　　　*Phosphorus: 80mg*

Protein: 4 grams　　　　　　　　　 *Sodium: 30mg*

Potassium: 100mg (depending on berry type)

TIPS FOR MODIFICATION:

- For lower potassium: Choose berries lower in potassium like blueberries or raspberries instead of mixed berries.
- For phosphorus control: Skip the walnuts or use a smaller amount as nuts are higher in phosphorus. You can substitute with a sprinkle of ground flaxseed for added fiber.

Scrambled Eggs with Bell Peppers and Mushrooms

Enjoy a protein boost without overloading your kidneys with this low-protein take on scrambled eggs. Bell peppers and mushrooms add flavor and essential nutrients, making it a satisfying and balanced CKD breakfast.

PREP TIME: 5 MINUTES | COOK TIME: 10 MINUTES | YIELDS: 1 SERVING

INGREDIENTS:

- 1 egg white
- ½ cup chopped red bell pepper
- ½ cup chopped mushrooms
- 1 teaspoon olive oil
- Salt-free herb seasoning (to taste)

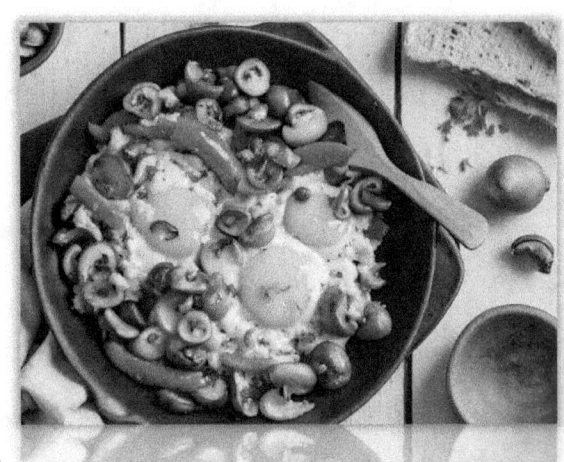

COOKING INSTRUCTIONS:

1. In a non-stick pan, heat olive oil over medium heat.
2. Add bell peppers and mushrooms, cook for 3-4 minutes, or until softened.
3. Push vegetables to the side of the pan. Add egg white and scramble until cooked through, about 2-3 minutes.
4. Season with salt-free herb seasoning to taste and enjoy!

NUTRITIONAL INFORMATION: (APPROXIMATE VALUES PER SERVING)

Calories: 120

Protein: 4 grams

Potassium: 150mg (depending on bell pepper variety)

Phosphorus: 80mg

Sodium: 40mg (depending on seasoning)

TIPS FOR MODIFICATION:

- For lower potassium: Choose green bell peppers instead of red, as they are lower in potassium.
- Sodium control: opt for a pre-washed and chopped option for bell peppers to minimize added sodium. You can also use a smaller amount of salt-free seasoning based on your taste preference.

Creamy Breakfast Polenta with Stewed Blackberries

Indulge in a warm and comforting breakfast without compromising your CKD diet. This recipe features creamy polenta topped with a low-potassium, low-phosphorus stewed blackberry compote, making it a delicious and kidney-friendly option.

PREP TIME: 5 MINUTES | COOK TIME: 20 MINUTES | YIELDS: 1 SERVING

INGREDIENTS:

- ½ cup rolled polenta
- 1 cup unsweetened almond milk
- ½ cup water
- ¼ teaspoon ground cinnamon
- ½ cup fresh or frozen blackberries
- 1 tablespoon water (for stewing)
- 1 teaspoon sugar substitute (optional)

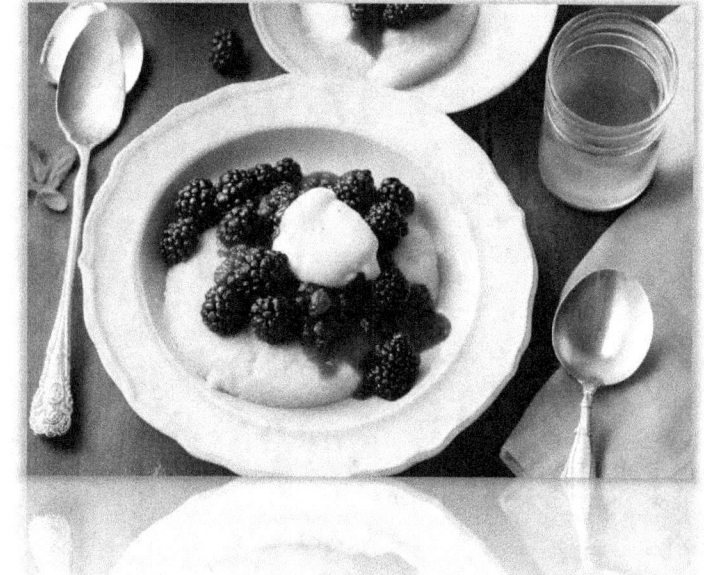

COOKING INSTRUCTIONS:

1. In a saucepan, whisk together polenta, almond milk, water, and cinnamon. Bring to a boil over medium heat.
2. Reduce heat to low and simmer for 15 minutes, or until polenta is cooked through and creamy, stirring occasionally.
3. While the polenta cooks, in a separate small saucepan, combine blackberries and 1 tablespoon of water. Cook over medium heat for 5-7 minutes, or until the berries soften and release their juices. You can mash some of the berries for a thicker consistency (optional).
4. If desired, stir in sugar substitute to the stewed blackberries (optional).
5. Pour cooked polenta into a bowl and top with the warmed stewed blackberries. Enjoy!

NUTRITIONAL INFORMATION: (APPROXIMATE VALUES PER SERVING)

Calories: 250

Protein: 4 grams

Phosphorus: 80mg

Potassium: 100mg (depending on blackberry ripeness)

Sodium: 30mg

TIPS FOR MODIFICATION:

- For lower potassium: Choose a smaller amount of blackberries or use a mix of berries with lower potassium content, like blueberries or raspberries.
- Phosphorus control: Skip the sugar substitute or use a very minimal amount. You can add a sprinkle of ground cinnamon for extra flavor without added phosphorus.

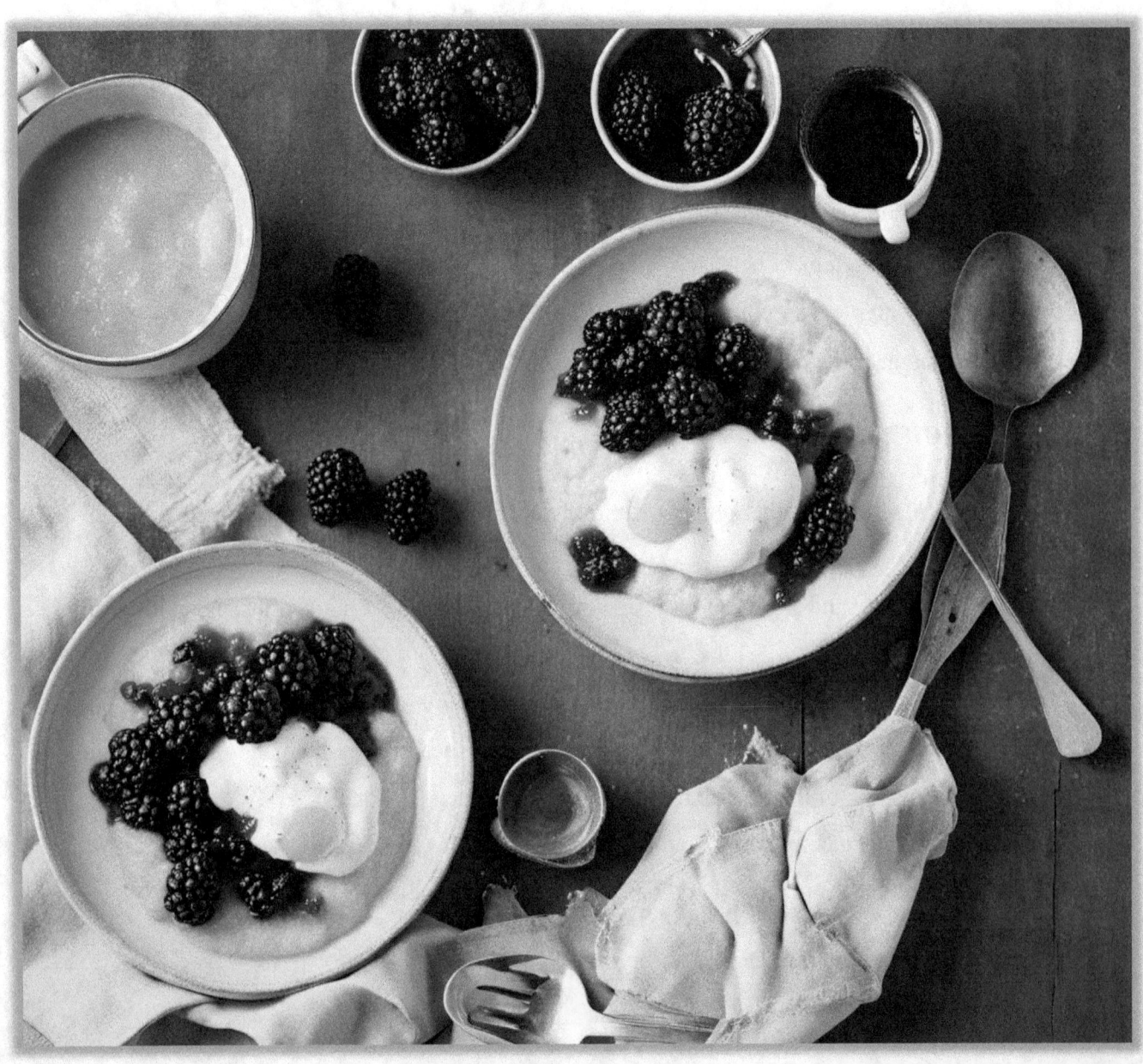

Huevo Ranchero (CKD-Friendly Omelet)

Enjoy a twist on the classic Huevo Ranchero with this kidney-friendly version. This recipe uses egg whites and low-potassium vegetables for a protein-packed omelet with a flavorful pepper and onion hash.

PREP TIME: 10 MINUTES | COOK TIME: 15 MINUTES | YIELDS: 1 SERVING

INGREDIENTS:

- 2 egg whites
- ½ cup chopped bell pepper (green or yellow recommended for lower potassium)
- ¼ cup chopped onion
- 1 tablespoon olive oil
- Salt-free herb seasoning (to taste)
- 1 tablespoon chopped fresh cilantro (optional)
- Salsa (low-sodium option)

COOKING INSTRUCTIONS:

1. In a non-stick pan, heat olive oil over medium heat.
2. Add chopped onion and cook for 2 minutes, or until softened.
3. Add chopped bell pepper and cook for an additional 3-4 minutes, or until tender-crisp.
4. Push the vegetables to the side of the pan. Add egg whites and scramble until cooked through, about 2-3 minutes.
5. Season with salt-free herb seasoning to taste.
6. Fold the vegetable hash over the scrambled egg whites.
7. Sprinkle with chopped fresh cilantro (optional) and serve immediately with your favorite low-sodium salsa.

NUTRITIONAL INFORMATION: (APPROXIMATE VALUES PER SERVING)

Calories: 200

Potassium: 150mg (depending on pepper variety)

Protein: 6 grams

Phosphorus: 80mg

Sodium: 40mg (depending on seasoning and salsa)

TIPS FOR MODIFICATION:

- For even lower potassium: Choose green or yellow bell peppers over red peppers, as they are generally lower in potassium.
- Sodium control: opt for a pre-washed and chopped option for bell peppers to minimize added sodium. You can also use a smaller amount of salt-free seasoning based on your taste preference.

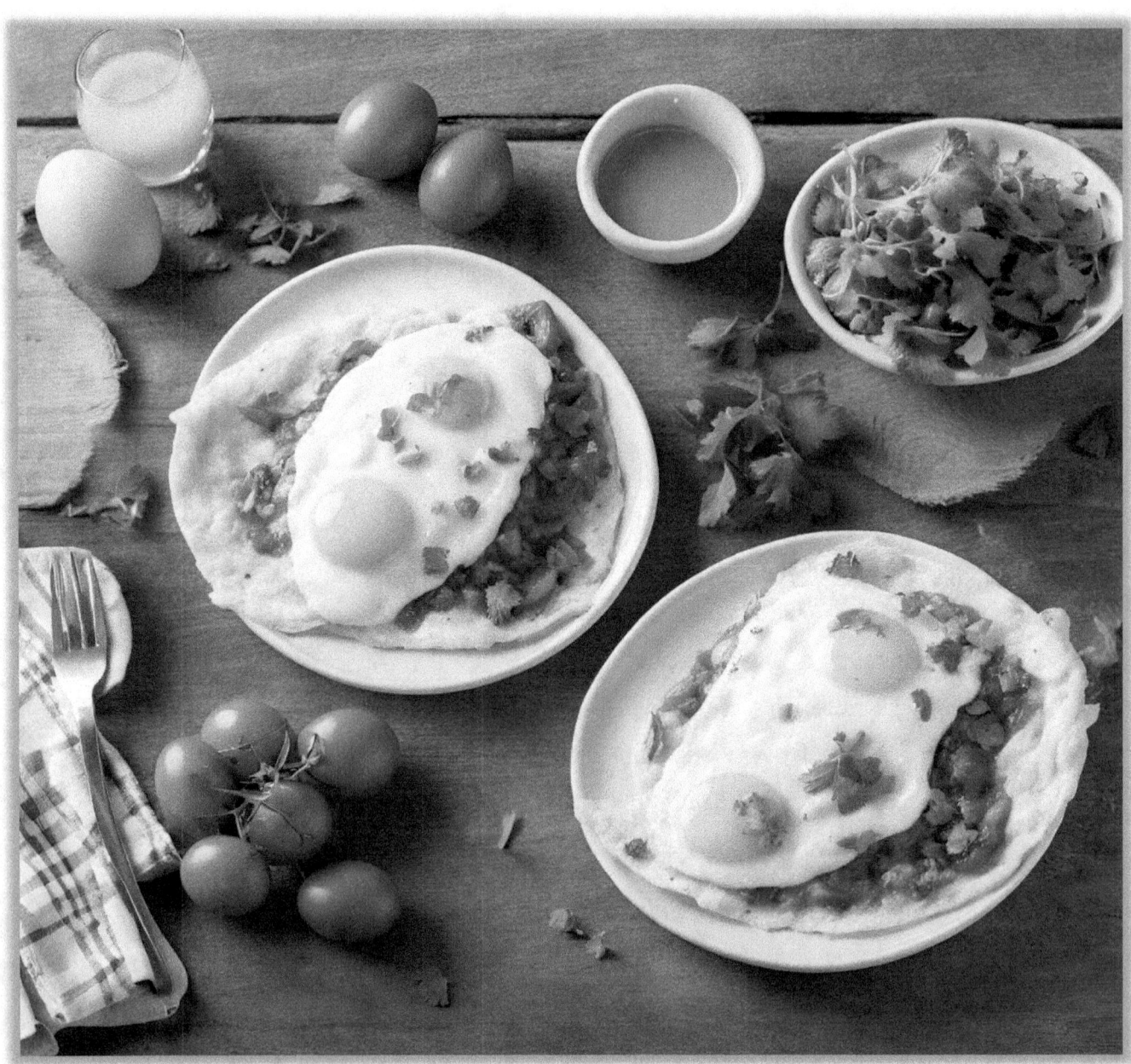

Shakshuka

Enjoy a flavorful and protein-boosted breakfast without straining your kidneys! This CKD-friendly shakshuka uses egg whites and swaps traditional high-potassium ingredients for lower-potassium alternatives, making it a delicious and kidney-friendly option.

PREP TIME: 5 MINUTES | COOK TIME: 15 MINUTES | YIELDS: 1 SERVING

INGREDIENTS:

- 2 egg whites
- ½ cup chopped tomatoes (diced canned tomatoes with no added salt recommended)
- ¼ cup chopped mushrooms
- ¼ cup chopped onion
- 1 tablespoon olive oil
- ½ teaspoon paprika
- Salt-free herb seasoning (to taste)

COOKING INSTRUCTIONS:

1. In a non-stick pan, heat olive oil over medium heat.
2. Add chopped onion and cook for 2 minutes, or until softened.
3. Add chopped mushrooms and cook for an additional 2 minutes, or until tender.
4. Add diced tomatoes and paprika. Season with a pinch of salt-free herb seasoning (optional). Simmer for 5 minutes to let the flavors meld.
5. Create two wells in the tomato mixture. Crack an egg white into each well.
6. Cover the pan and cook for 3-4 minutes, or until the egg whites are set.
7. Season with additional salt-free herb seasoning to taste and enjoy!

NUTRITIONAL INFORMATION: (APPROXIMATE VALUES PER SERVING)

Calories: 200

Phosphorus: 80mg

Protein: 6 grams

Sodium: 40mg (depending on seasoning)

Potassium: 200mg (depending on tomato type)

TIPS FOR MODIFICATION:

- For lower potassium: Use low-potassium canned tomatoes with no added salt. You can also rinse canned tomatoes before adding them to the dish.
- Phosphorus control: Skip adding cheese or use a very minimal amount of low-phosphorus cheese alternative specifically designed for CKD diets.

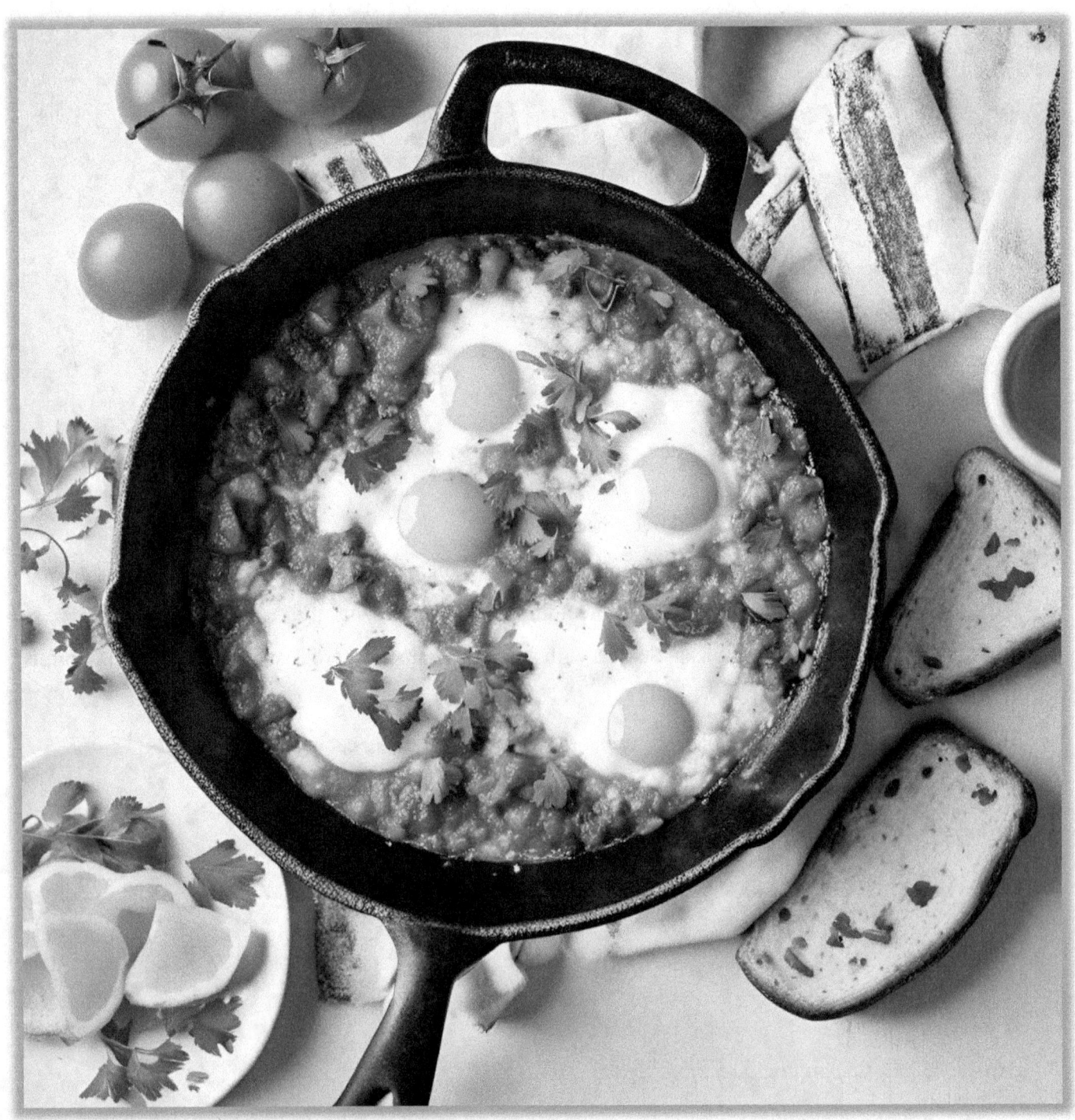

Pecan and Fruit Bowls

This delightful bowl combines the satisfying crunch of pecans with a refreshing medley of fruits. Packed with fiber and low in protein, potassium, and phosphorus, it's a delicious and kidney-friendly way to start your day or enjoy a satisfying snack.

PREP TIME: 5 MINUTES | COOK TIME: NO COOK TIME | YIELDS: 1 SERVING

INGREDIENTS:

- ½ cup chopped mixed fruits (choose from berries, melon, or chopped apple)
- ¼ cup chopped pecans
- 1 tablespoon plain low-fat yogurt (optional)
- ¼ teaspoon ground cinnamon

COOKING INSTRUCTIONS:

1. In a bowl, combine chopped fruits and pecans.
2. Top with a dollop of plain low-fat yogurt (optional).
3. Sprinkle with ground cinnamon and enjoy!

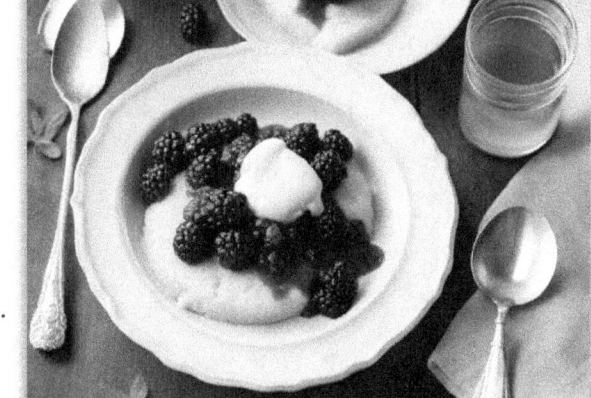

NUTRITIONAL INFORMATION: (APPROXIMATE VALUES PER SERVING)

Calories: 200

Phosphorus: 80mg

Protein: 2 grams (depending on yogurt)

Sodium: 30mg (depending on yogurt)

Potassium: 150mg (depending on fruit choices)

TIPS FOR MODIFICATION:

- For lower potassium: Choose fruits lower in potassium like blueberries, raspberries, or chopped Granny Smith apples.
- Protein control: Skip the yogurt or use a smaller amount. You can substitute with a sprinkle of ground flaxseed for added fiber.

Green Pineapple Smoothie

Enjoy a refreshing and kidney-friendly twist on a classic green smoothie! This recipe uses low-potassium and low-phosphorus greens paired with the sweetness of pineapple for a delicious and balanced breakfast or snack.

PREP TIME: 5 MINUTES | COOK TIME: NO COOK TIME | YIELDS: 1 SERVING

INGREDIENTS:

- 1 cup unsweetened almond milk
- ½ cup frozen pineapple chunks
- ½ cup chopped spinach or kale (depending on preference)
- ¼ cup chopped cucumber
- ¼ avocado (optional)
- Handful of ice cubes

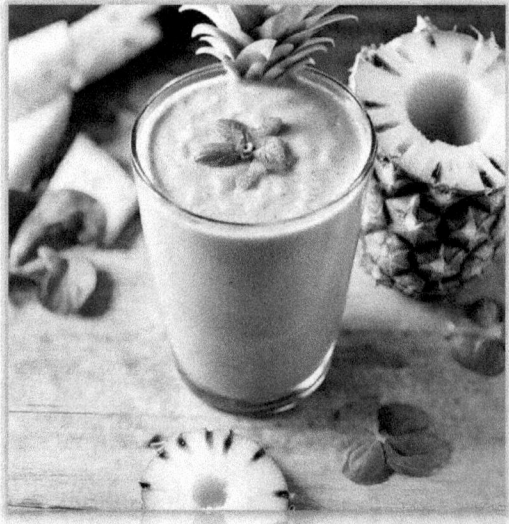

COOKING INSTRUCTIONS:

1. Combine all ingredients in a blender and blend until smooth and creamy.
2. Enjoy immediately!

NUTRITIONAL INFORMATION: (APPROXIMATE VALUES PER SERVING)

Calories: 200

Phosphorus: 80mg

Protein: 1 gram (depending on avocado)

Sodium: 30mg

Potassium: 200mg (depending on greens)

TIPS FOR MODIFICATION:

- For lower potassium: Choose spinach over kale as it's generally lower in potassium.
- Phosphorus control: Skip the avocado or use a very minimal amount. You can substitute with a scoop of low-phosphorus protein powder (if allowed in your diet) for added protein.

Cottage Cheese with Pineapple and Papaya

This refreshing and light breakfast is perfect for those on a CKD diet. Packed with protein from cottage cheese and balanced by the sweetness of pineapple and papaya, it's a delicious way to start your day without straining your kidneys.

PREP TIME: 5 MINUTES | COOK TIME: 0 MINUTES | YIELDS: 1 SERVING

INGREDIENTS:

- ½ cup low-fat cottage cheese
- ½ cup diced fresh pineapple
- ¼ cup diced papaya
- 1 tablespoon chopped mint (optional)

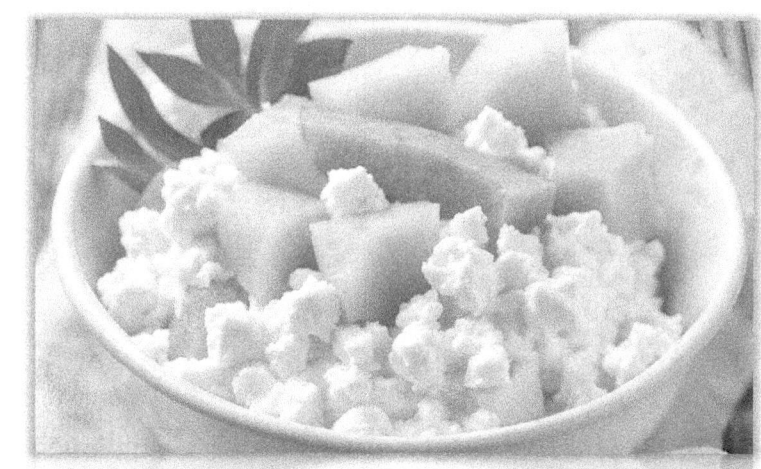

COOKING INSTRUCTIONS:

1. In a bowl, combine cottage cheese, diced pineapple, and diced papaya.
2. Garnish with chopped mint (optional) and enjoy!

NUTRITIONAL INFORMATION: (APPROXIMATE VALUES PER SERVING)

Calories: 150

Phosphorus: 150mg

Protein: 12 grams

Sodium: 80mg

Potassium: 200mg (depending on fruit ripeness)

TIPS FOR MODIFICATION:

- For lower potassium: Use a slightly smaller amount of pineapple and papaya, opting for more towards the pineapple as it's generally lower in potassium.
- Potassium control: If potassium is a major concern, consider substituting berries such as blueberries or raspberries for the pineapple and papaya.

High-Fiber Cereal with Berries

Get a satisfying and fiber-filled start to your day with this CKD-friendly cereal recipe. Low in protein, potassium, and phosphorus, it keeps you feeling full while supporting your kidney health.

PREP TIME: 2 MINUTES | COOK TIME: (DEPENDS ON CEREAL COOKING INSTRUCTIONS) | YIELDS: 1 SERVING

INGREDIENTS:

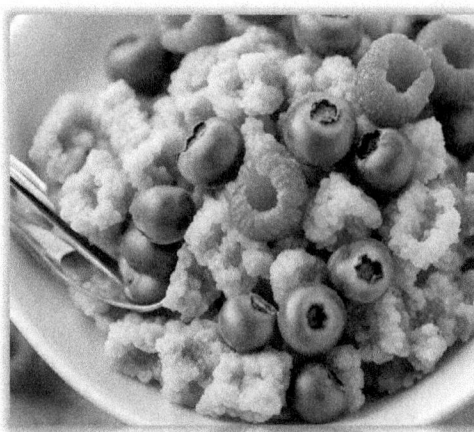

- ¾ cup shredded wheat cereal (check for low-sodium options)
- 1 cup unsweetened almond milk
- ½ cup mixed berries
- 2 tablespoons chopped almonds

COOKING INSTRUCTIONS:

1. Follow the package instructions to cook the cereal (usually boiling water for a few minutes).
2. Pour cooked cereal into a bowl and add unsweetened almond milk.
3. Top with mixed berries and chopped almonds. Enjoy!

NUTRITIONAL INFORMATION: (APPROXIMATE VALUES PER SERVING)

Calories: 250

Phosphorus: 100mg

Protein: 5 grams

Sodium: 40mg (depending on cereal choice)

Potassium: 150mg (depending on berry type)

TIPS FOR MODIFICATION:

- For lower potassium: Choose berries lower in potassium like blueberries or raspberries instead of mixed berries.
- Phosphorus control: Skip the almonds or use a smaller amount. You can substitute with a sprinkle of ground flaxseed for added fiber.

Baked Sweet Potato with Chia Seeds

This simple recipe transforms a sweet potato into a delicious and nutritious breakfast option for CKD patients. Packed with fiber and low in protein, potassium, and phosphorus, it's a satisfying and kidney-friendly way to start your day.

PREP TIME: 5 MINUTES | COOK TIME: 45 MINUTES | YIELDS: 1 SERVING

INGREDIENTS:

- 1 small sweet potato
- 2 tablespoons plain low-fat yogurt
- 1 tablespoon chia seeds
- ¼ teaspoon ground cinnamon

COOKING INSTRUCTIONS:

1. Preheat oven to 400°F (200°C). Wash and pierce the sweet potato with a fork a few times.
2. Place the sweet potato directly on the oven rack and bake for 45 minutes, or until tender when pierced with a fork.
3. While the sweet potato bakes, in a small bowl, combine yogurt, chia seeds, and cinnamon.
4. Once the sweet potato is cooked, let it cool slightly before cutting it open.
5. Top the sweet potato with the yogurt-chia seed mixture and enjoy!

NUTRITIONAL INFORMATION: (APPROXIMATE VALUES PER SERVING)

Calories: 200

Phosphorus: 80mg

Protein: 3 grams

Sodium: 30mg

Potassium: 200mg

TIPS FOR MODIFICATION:

- For lower potassium: Choose a smaller sweet potato as they tend to have lower potassium content.
- Potassium and Phosphorus control: If potassium and phosphorus are a major concern, consider substituting the yogurt with a small amount of low-potassium and low-phosphorus fruit like diced apples or berries.

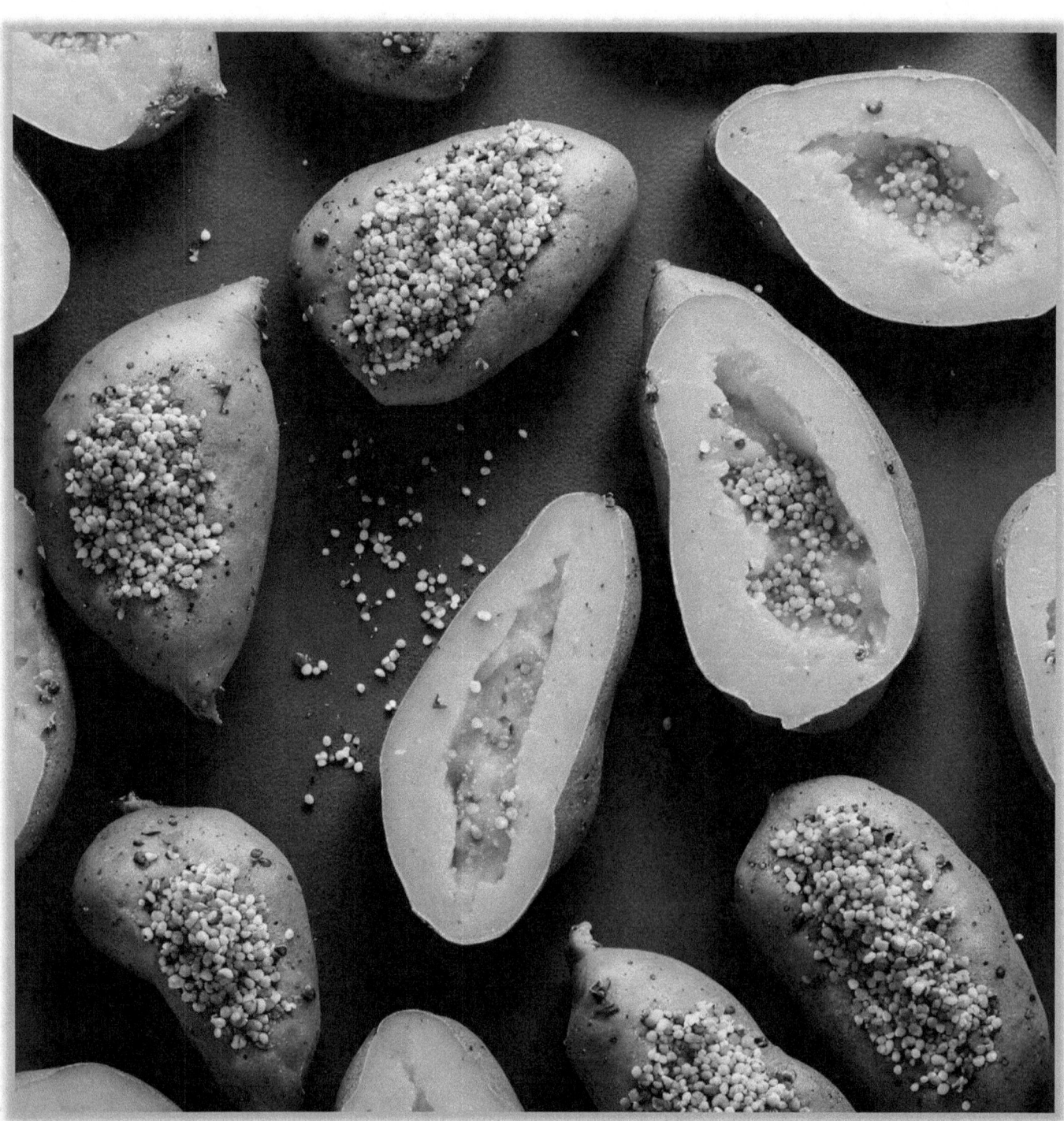

Pear and Ricotta Toast

This simple toast recipe offers a delightful balance of sweetness and creaminess. Perfect for CKD patients, it's low in protein, potassium, and phosphorus, making it a delicious and kidney-friendly breakfast option.

PREP TIME: 5 MINUTES | COOK TIME: (DEPENDS ON TOASTING PREFERENCE) | YIELDS: 1 SERVING

INGREDIENTS:

- 1 slice whole-wheat toast
- 2 tablespoons low-fat ricotta cheese
- ½ pear, thinly sliced
- Sprinkle of ground cinnamon

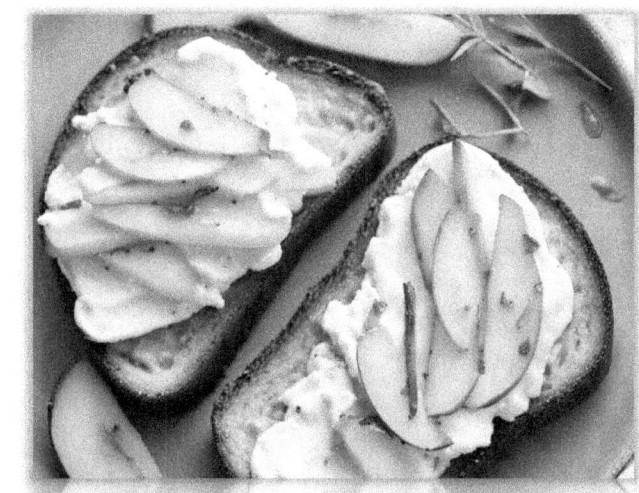

COOKING INSTRUCTIONS:

1. Toast your bread to your desired level of doneness.
2. Spread ricotta cheese evenly over the toast.
3. Arrange thinly sliced pear on top of the ricotta cheese.
4. Sprinkle with ground cinnamon and enjoy!

NUTRITIONAL INFORMATION: (APPROXIMATE VALUES PER SERVING)

Calories: 180

Phosphorus: 80mg

Protein: 4 grams

Sodium: 60mg

Potassium: 150mg (depending on pear variety)

TIPS FOR MODIFICATION:

- For lower potassium: Choose pear varieties lower in potassium like Asian pears compared to Bartlett pears.
- Protein control: If protein is a major concern, opt for a single tablespoon of ricotta cheese or a low-protein ricotta alternative.

Low-Sodium Breakfast Burrito

Start your day with a satisfying and portable breakfast without the added sodium. This recipe uses low-sodium ingredients and skips processed meats, making it a delicious and kidney-friendly option for Stage 3 CKD patients.

PREP TIME: 10 MINUTES | COOK TIME: 5 MINUTES (DEPENDING ON SCRAMBLED EGG PREFERENCE) | YIELDS: 1 SERVING

INGREDIENTS:

- 1 whole-wheat tortilla
- 1 scrambled egg white
- ¼ cup chopped black beans (rinsed and drained)
- 2 tablespoons shredded low-sodium cheese
- Salsa (low-sodium option)

COOKING INSTRUCTIONS:

1. Scramble one egg white using a small amount of non-stick cooking spray. Season with salt-free herb seasoning (optional).
2. Warm a whole-wheat tortilla in a dry pan or microwave for a few seconds to make it pliable.
3. Spread the scrambled egg white onto the tortilla.
4. Top with chopped black beans, shredded low-sodium cheese, and a dollop of low-sodium salsa.
5. Fold the bottom of the tortilla up and over the filling, then fold in the sides. Roll up tightly to create a burrito.

NUTRITIONAL INFORMATION: (APPROXIMATE VALUES PER SERVING)

Calories: 250

Potassium: 200mg (depending on salsa)

Protein: 7 grams

Phosphorus: 150mg

Sodium: 150mg (depending on salsa choice)

<u>TIPS FOR MODIFICATION:</u>

- For lower potassium: Choose black beans that have been canned with low-sodium or no added salt. You can also rinse them thoroughly before using to remove some of the potassium content.
- Phosphorus control: opt for a smaller amount of cheese or choose a low-phosphorus cheese alternative specifically made for CKD diets.

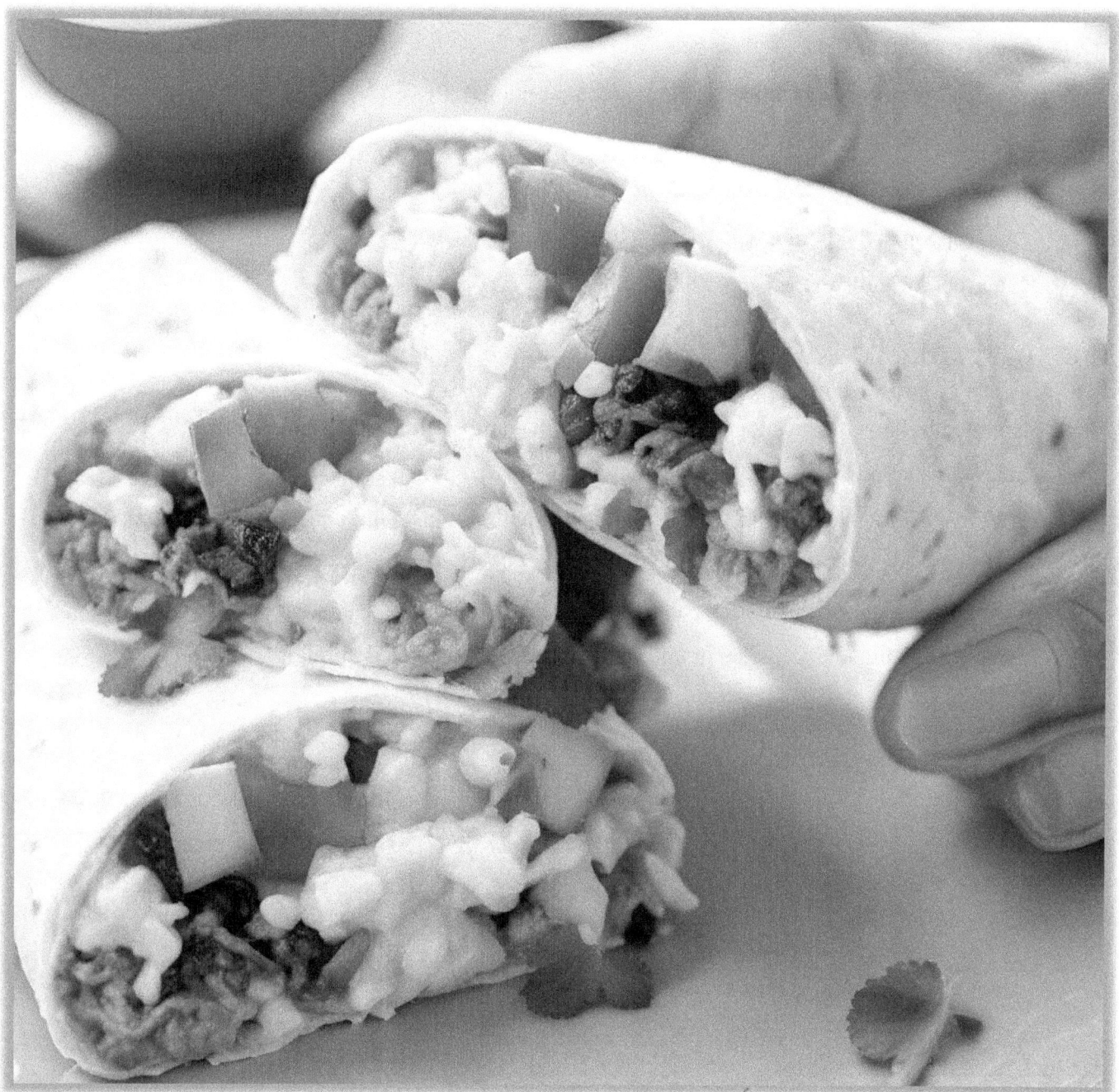

Protein-Free Pancakes

Enjoy fluffy pancakes without the protein! This recipe uses clever modifications to minimize protein content, making it a delicious and kidney-friendly option for those on a low-protein CKD diet.

PREP TIME: 5 MINUTES | COOK TIME: 10 MINUTES | YIELDS: 2 SMALL PANCAKES

INGREDIENTS:

- ¾ cup cornstarch
- ¼ cup all-purpose flour (check for low-sodium options)
- 1 tablespoon sugar substitute
- 1 cup unsweetened almond milk
- 1 tablespoon melted butter
- ½ teaspoon vanilla extract

COOKING INSTRUCTIONS:

1. In a medium bowl, whisk together cornstarch, all-purpose flour, and sugar substitute.
2. In a separate bowl, whisk together almond milk, melted butter, and vanilla extract.
3. Pour the wet ingredients into the dry ingredients and mix just until combined (a few lumps are okay).
4. Heat a lightly greased non-stick pan over medium heat. Pour ¼ cup batter per pancake.
5. Cook for 2-3 minutes per side, or until golden brown and cooked through.
6. Serve immediately and enjoy!

NUTRITIONAL INFORMATION: (APPROXIMATE VALUES PER PANCAKE)

Calories: 100

Phosphorus: 60mg

Protein: 1 gram (very low)

Sodium: 40mg (depending on milk type)

Potassium: 30mg (depending on milk type)

TIPS FOR MODIFICATION:

- For further phosphorus reduction: Consider using a low-phosphorus flour alternative specifically designed for CKD diets.
- Sodium control: Use low-sodium milk or lactose-free milk options to minimize sodium intake.

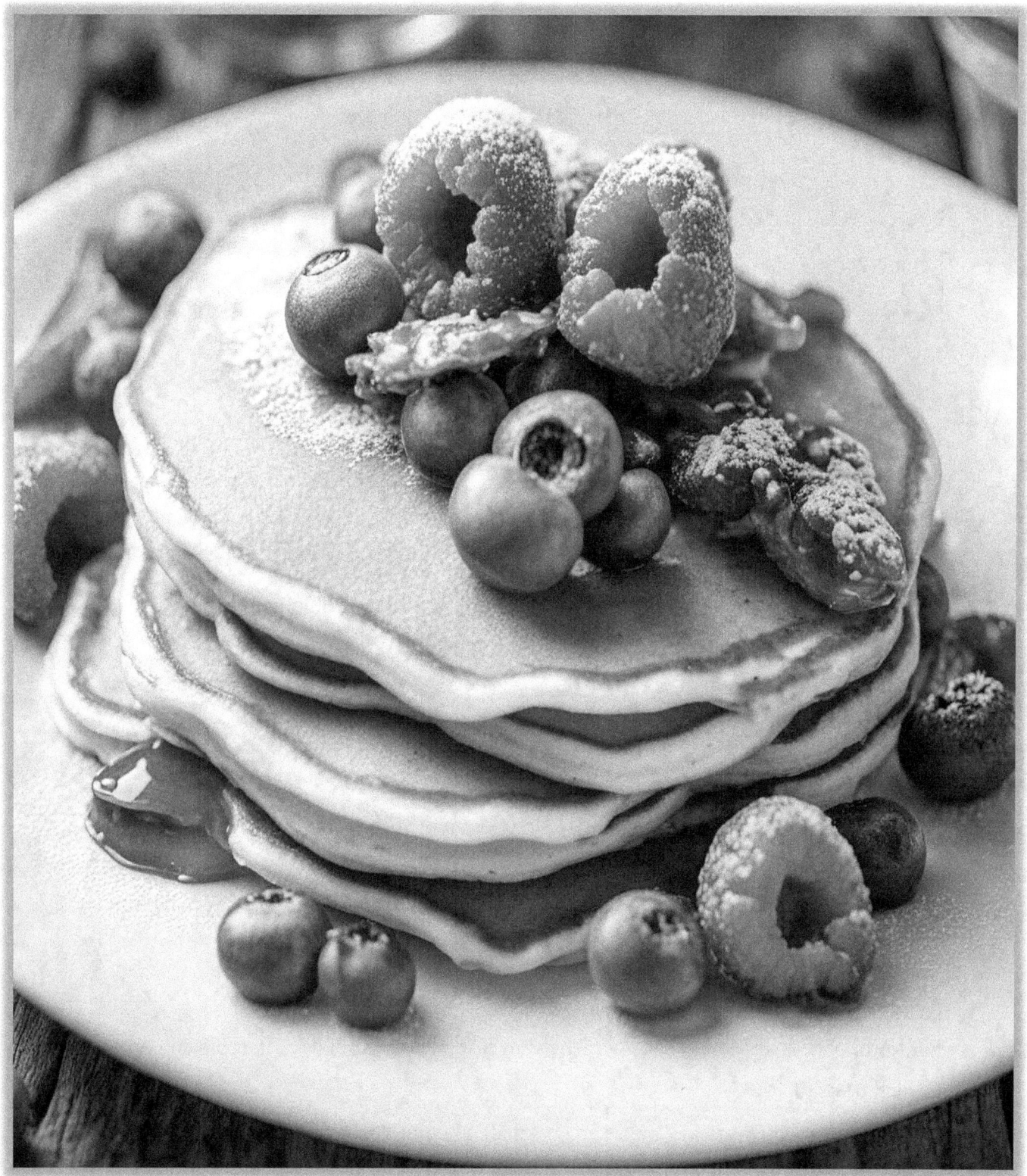

Poached Pears with Ginger

Warm up your mornings with this comforting and kidney-friendly dessert. Poached pears infused with ginger create a delightful and low-protein, low-potassium, and low-phosphorus treat.

PREP TIME: 5 MINUTES | COOK TIME: 15 MINUTES | YIELDS: 1 SERVING

INGREDIENTS:

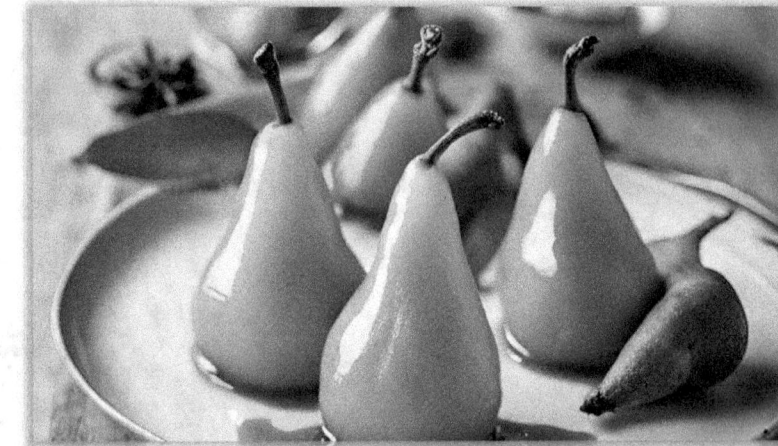

- 2 pears, peeled and cored
- 1 cup water
- 1 tablespoon chopped fresh ginger
- 1 teaspoon honey (optional)

COOKING INSTRUCTIONS:

1. In a saucepan, combine water and chopped ginger. Bring to a simmer over medium heat.
2. Gently add the pears and simmer for 10-15 minutes, or until the pears are tender when pierced with a fork.
3. Remove from heat and let the pears cool slightly in the poaching liquid.
4. Transfer the pears to a bowl. Drizzle with a little poaching liquid and top with honey (optional).

NUTRITIONAL INFORMATION: (APPROXIMATE VALUES PER SERVING)

Calories: 150

Phosphorus: 30mg

Protein: 1 gram

Sodium: 10mg

Potassium: 150mg (depending on pear variety)

TIPS FOR MODIFICATION:

- For lower potassium: Choose pear varieties lower in potassium like Asian pears compared to Bartlett pears.
- Sugar control: Skip the honey or use a very small amount. You can substitute with a few sugar substitute drops for a touch of sweetness without added potassium.

LUNCH RECIPES

Welcome to Kidney-Friendly Lunch Recipes

Lunchtime is an opportunity to nourish your body with a meal that keeps your energy levels steady and supports your kidney health. The lunch recipes in this section are crafted specifically for individuals like YOU managing Stage 3 kidney disease. Each recipe focuses on being low in protein, potassium, sodium, and phosphorus, making them both safe and delicious.

In this collection, you'll find a variety of vibrant and flavorful dishes that highlight fresh vegetables, unique seasonings, and kidney-friendly ingredients. From the aromatic Vegetable Masala to the refreshing Thai Pineapple Salad with Carrot Cashew Dressing, these recipes are designed to provide a satisfying and nutrient-rich meal without compromising your dietary needs.

What to Expect

1. Flavorful and Aromatic Dishes: Recipes like Vegetable Masala and Gumbo Z'Herbes offer rich flavors using kidney-friendly spices and herbs.
2. Refreshing and Light Options: Enjoy light and refreshing meals such as the Thai Pineapple Salad with Carrot Cashew Dressing and Beet Salad with Candied or Spiced Pecans.
3. Comforting Soups and Hearty Meals: Find comfort in dishes like Pumpkin Soup with "Chorizo" Mushrooms and Corn, and Corn and Chile Soup with Smoky Collard Greens.
4. Versatile Vinaigrettes: Learn to prepare versatile dressings like Lemon-Herb Vinaigrette and Curry-Ginger Vinaigrette to enhance the flavors of your salads and side dishes.
5. Nutritious and Satisfying Options: Recipes like the Tostada Salad and Baked Sweet Potato with Side Salad offer a balanced and satisfying meal that supports kidney health.
6. By incorporating these lunch recipes into your daily routine, you can enjoy a diverse and delicious range of meals that align with your dietary needs for Stage 3 kidney disease. Each recipe is designed to be easy to follow and full of flavor, making lunchtime a delightful and nutritious part of your day.

Vegetable Masala

Spice up your lunch routine with this vibrant and flavorful vegetable masala! Packed with low-protein, low-potassium, and low-phosphorus vegetables, it's a delicious and kidney-friendly option that will keep you satisfied.

PREP TIME: 10 MINUTES | COOK TIME: 20 MINUTES | YIELDS: 1 SERVING

INGREDIENTS:

- 1 tablespoon olive oil
- ½ cup chopped onion
- ½ cup chopped bell pepper (green or yellow recommended)
- ½ cup chopped zucchini
- ¼ cup chopped tomatoes (diced canned tomatoes with no added salt recommended)
- 1 teaspoon curry powder
- ½ teaspoon ground cumin
- ½ cup vegetable broth (low-sodium option)
- Salt-free herb seasoning (to taste)
- Cilantro (optional, for garnish)

COOKING INSTRUCTIONS:

1. In a saucepan, heat olive oil over medium heat.
2. Add chopped onion and cook for 2-3 minutes, or until softened.
3. Add chopped bell pepper and zucchini, cook for an additional 3-4 minutes, or until tender-crisp.
4. Stir in diced tomatoes, curry powder, and cumin. Season with a pinch of salt-free herb seasoning (optional).
5. Pour in vegetable broth and bring to a simmer. Cook for 5-7 minutes, or until the vegetables are softened and flavors are combined.
6. Adjust seasonings with additional salt-free herb seasoning to taste.
7. Serve hot, garnished with fresh cilantro (optional).

NUTRITIONAL INFORMATION: (APPROXIMATE VALUES PER SERVING)

Calories: 200 *Phosphorus: 100mg*

Protein: 2 grams *Sodium: 40mg (depending on seasoning and broth*

Potassium: 250mg (depending on vegetables)

)

TIPS FOR MODIFICATION:

- For even lower potassium: Choose green or yellow bell peppers over red peppers, as they tend to be lower in potassium. You can also rinse canned tomatoes before adding them.
- Phosphorus control: opt for a pre-washed and chopped option for vegetables to minimize added sodium. You can also use a smaller amount of vegetable broth and adjust the consistency with water.

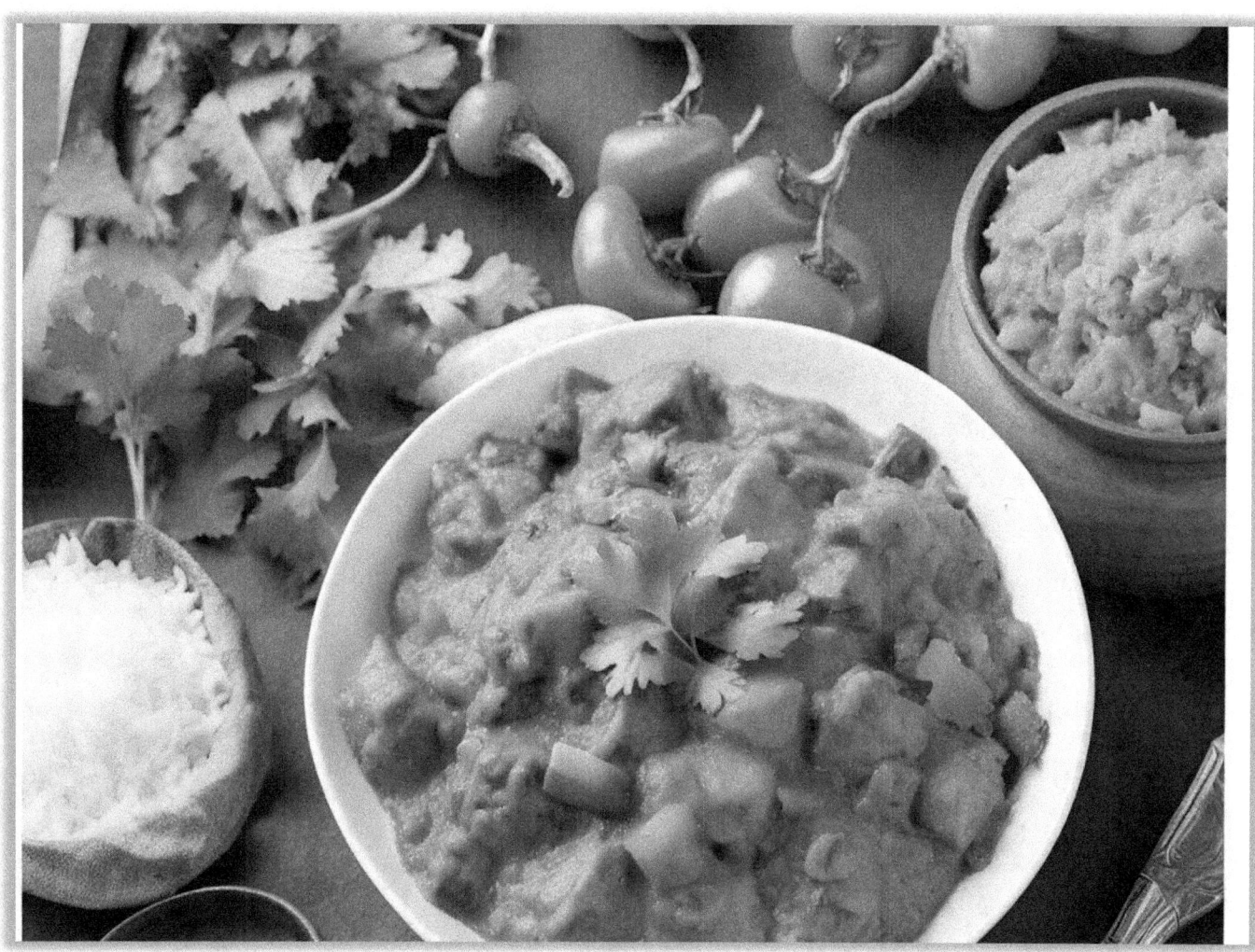

Gumbo Z'Herbes

This lighter take on the classic Gumbo Z'Herbes offers a vibrant and flavorful lunch option for those on a CKD diet. Packed with low-protein greens and a vegetable-based roux, it provides a satisfying and kidney-friendly meal.

PREP TIME: 15 MINUTES | COOK TIME: 30 MINUTES | YIELDS: 1 SERVING

INGREDIENTS:

- ½ tablespoon olive oil
- ½ cup chopped onion
- ½ cup chopped celery
- ½ cup chopped turnips (peeled and chopped)
- 1 cup chopped turnip greens or collard greens (rinsed and chopped)
- 1 cup vegetable broth (low-sodium option)
- 1 tablespoon whole wheat flour
- 1 teaspoon Worcestershire sauce (low-sodium option)
- Salt-free herb seasoning (to taste)
- Hot sauce (optional, for garnish)

COOKING INSTRUCTIONS:

1. In a large pot, heat olive oil over medium heat.
2. Add chopped onion, celery, and turnips. Cook for 5 minutes, or until softened.
3. Stir in whole wheat flour and cook for an additional minute to create a light roux.
4. Pour in vegetable broth and bring to a simmer.
5. Add turnip greens or collard greens, Worcestershire sauce, and salt-free herb seasoning to taste.
6. Simmer for 20-25 minutes, or until the vegetables are tender and flavors are melded.
7. Adjust seasonings with additional salt-free herb seasoning if needed.
8. Serve hot with a sprinkle of hot sauce (optional).

NUTRITIONAL INFORMATION: (APPROXIMATE VALUES PER SERVING)

Calories: 250

Potassium: 300mg (depending on greens)

Protein: 4 grams

Phosphorus: 120mg

Sodium: 50mg (depending on broth and Worcestershire sauce)

TIPS FOR MODIFICATION:

- For lower potassium: Choose collard greens over turnip greens as they tend to be slightly lower in potassium. You can also cook the greens separately and add them towards the end for less potassium leaching.
- Phosphorus control: Skip adding Worcestershire sauce or use a very small amount of a low-sodium, phosphorus-conscious option. You can add a splash of lemon juice for extra flavor.

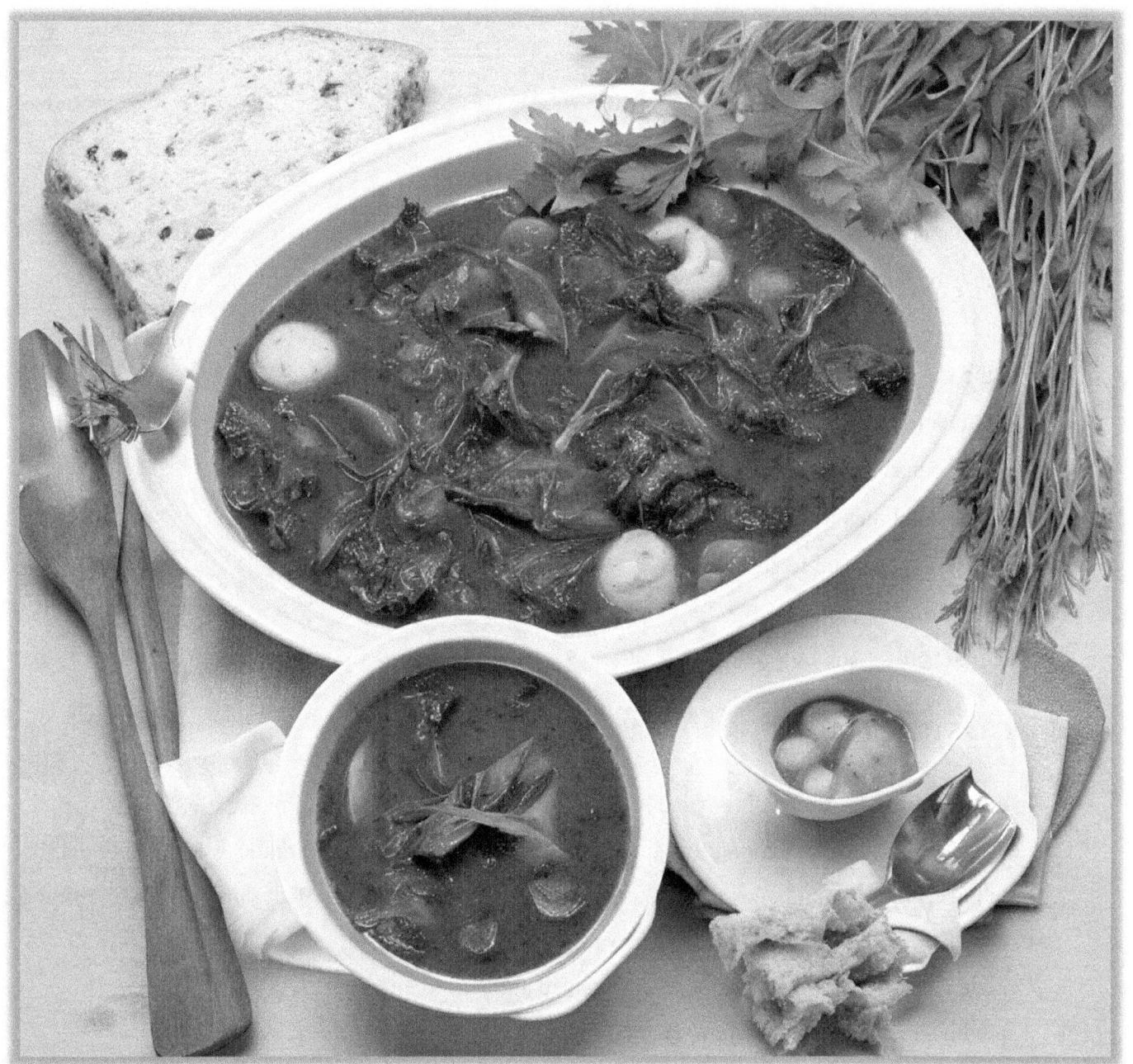

Thai Pineapple Salad with Carrot Cashew Dressing

Enjoy the sweet and savory flavors of Thailand with this refreshing and kidney-friendly salad! Packed with low-protein vegetables and a creamy cashew dressing made without added phosphorus, it's a delightful and satisfying lunch option for CKD patients.

PREP TIME: 15 MINUTES | COOK TIME: NO COOK TIME | YIELDS: 1 SERVING

INGREDIENTS:

- 1 cup chopped romaine lettuce
- ½ cup chopped cucumber
- ½ cup chopped bell pepper (any color)
- ½ cup chopped fresh pineapple
- ¼ cup chopped roasted cashews
- For the Carrot Cashew Dressing:
- 1 small carrot, peeled and grated
- 2 tablespoons unsweetened almond milk
- 1 tablespoon lime juice
- 1 tablespoon chopped fresh cilantro
- Pinch of ground ginger
- Salt-free herb seasoning (to taste)

COOKING INSTRUCTIONS:

1. In a bowl, combine chopped romaine lettuce, cucumber, bell pepper, and pineapple.
2. For the Carrot Cashew Dressing: In a blender or food processor, combine grated carrot, almond milk, lime juice, cilantro, and ginger. Blend until smooth and creamy. Season with salt-free herb seasoning to taste.
3. Drizzle the carrot cashew dressing over the salad and toss to coat.
4. Top with chopped roasted cashews and enjoy!

NUTRITIONAL INFORMATION: (APPROXIMATE VALUES PER SERVING)

Calories: 300

Phosphorus: 150mg (depending on cashews)

Protein: 4 grams (from cashews)

Sodium: 30mg (depending on seasoning)

Potassium: 200mg (depending on vegetables)

TIPS FOR MODIFICATION:

- For lower potassium: Choose green or yellow bell peppers over red peppers, as they tend to be lower in potassium.
- Phosphorus control: Limit the amount of cashews or use a smaller portion. You can substitute with chopped peanuts for a similar crunch (be mindful of allergies).

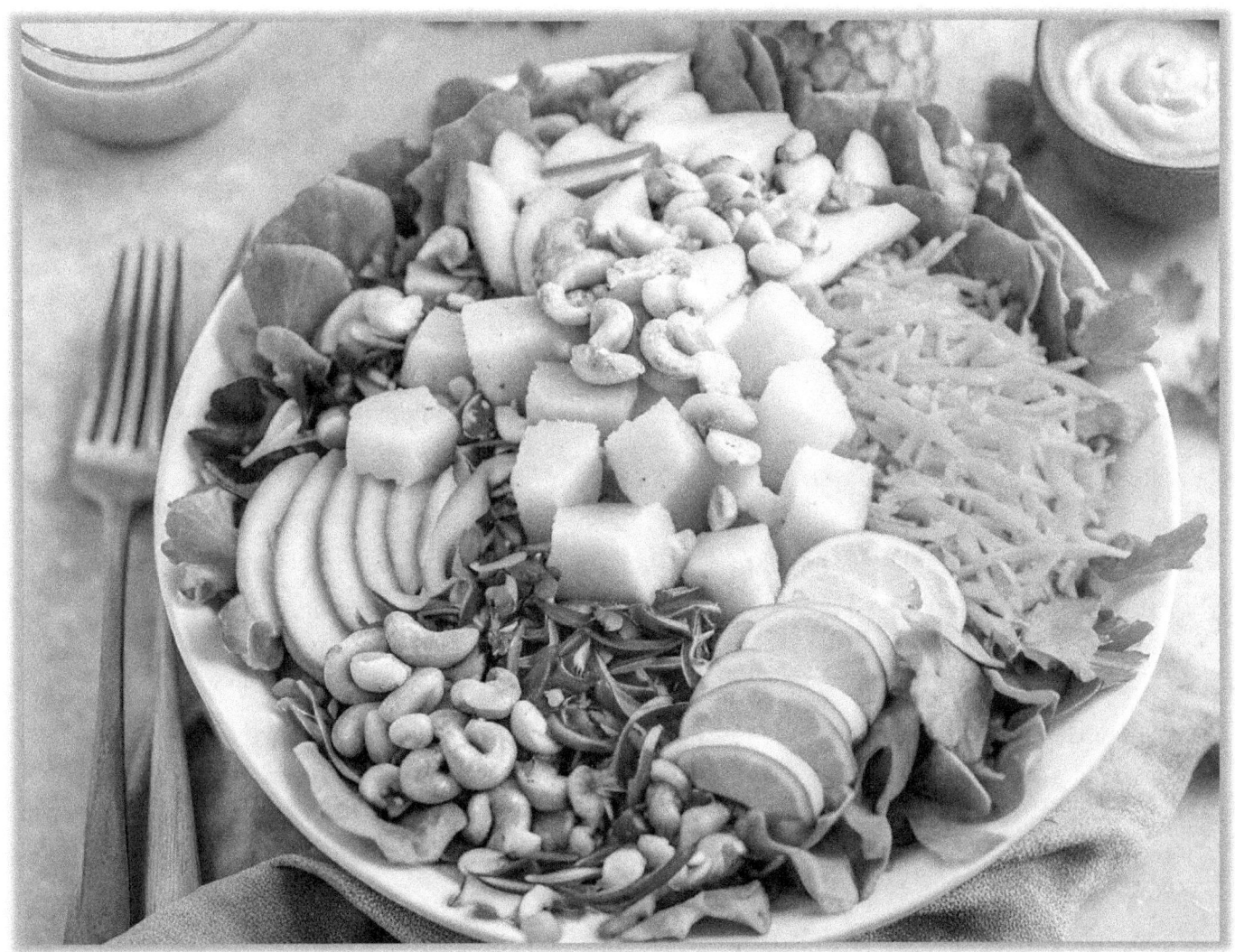

Lemon-Herb Vinaigrette

Dress up your CKD-friendly lunch salads with this flavorful and kidney-friendly vinaigrette! Made with simple ingredients and minimal phosphorus and potassium, it adds a bright and refreshing touch to your meal.

PREP TIME: 5 MINUTES | COOK TIME: NO COOK TIME | YIELDS: 1 SERVING

INGREDIENTS:

- 2 tablespoons olive oil
- 1 tablespoon lemon juice
- 1 teaspoon Dijon mustard (low-sodium option)
- ½ teaspoon dried oregano
- ¼ teaspoon dried thyme
- Pinch of garlic powder
- Salt-free herb seasoning (to taste)

COOKING INSTRUCTIONS:

1. In a small bowl, whisk together olive oil, lemon juice, Dijon mustard, oregano, thyme, and garlic powder.
2. Season with salt-free herb seasoning to taste.
3. Serve immediately or store in an airtight container in the refrigerator for up to a week.

NUTRITIONAL INFORMATION: (APPROXIMATE VALUES PER SERVING)

Calories: 100

Phosphorus: 10mg

Protein: 0 grams

Sodium: 30mg (depending on mustard)

Potassium: 30mg (depending on herbs)

TIPS FOR MODIFICATION:

- Minimize sodium: Choose a low-sodium Dijon mustard option to keep sodium intake in check.
- Fresh vs. dried herbs: You can substitute fresh herbs for dried herbs, but be mindful of portion sizes as they tend to be higher in potassium.

Pumpkin Soup with "Chorizo" Mushrooms and Corn

Enjoy the cozy flavors of fall with this delightful and kidney-friendly pumpkin soup! This recipe uses protein-free "chorizo" mushrooms and skips high-potassium ingredients for a satisfying and nourishing lunch option for CKD patients.

PREP TIME: 10 MINUTES | COOK TIME: 25 MINUTES | YIELDS: 1 SERVING

- INGREDIENTS:
- ½ tablespoon olive oil
- ½ cup chopped onion
- 1 clove garlic, minced
- ½ cup chopped "chorizo" mushrooms (or regular button mushrooms)
- 1 cup diced canned pumpkin (no added salt)
- 1 cup vegetable broth (low-sodium option)
- ¼ cup chopped corn (fresh or frozen)
- ½ teaspoon ground cumin
- ¼ teaspoon ground cinnamon
- Salt-free herb seasoning (to taste)

COOKING INSTRUCTIONS:

1. In a saucepan, heat olive oil over medium heat.
2. Add chopped onion and cook for 2-3 minutes, or until softened.
3. Add minced garlic and cook for an additional minute.
4. Stir in chopped "chorizo" mushrooms and cook until softened and slightly browned, about 5 minutes.
5. Add diced canned pumpkin, vegetable broth, corn, cumin, and cinnamon. Season with a pinch of salt-free herb seasoning (optional).
6. Bring to a simmer and cook for 15-20 minutes, or until the vegetables are tender.

7. Using an immersion blender or transferring to a blender, puree the soup until smooth. You can adjust the consistency with additional broth if desired.
8. Season with additional salt-free herb seasoning to taste and serve hot.

NUTRITIONAL INFORMATION: (APPROXIMATE VALUES PER SERVING)

Calories: 250

Phosphorus: 80mg

Protein: 1 gram (from mushrooms)

Sodium: 40mg (depending on broth)

Potassium: 200mg (depending on pumpkin)

TIPS FOR MODIFICATION:

- For lower potassium: Choose brands of canned pumpkin labeled as low-potassium or rinse canned pumpkin before using to remove some of the potassium content.
- Protein control: Skip using "chorizo" mushrooms if protein needs strict monitoring. You can substitute with regular button mushrooms for a similar texture.

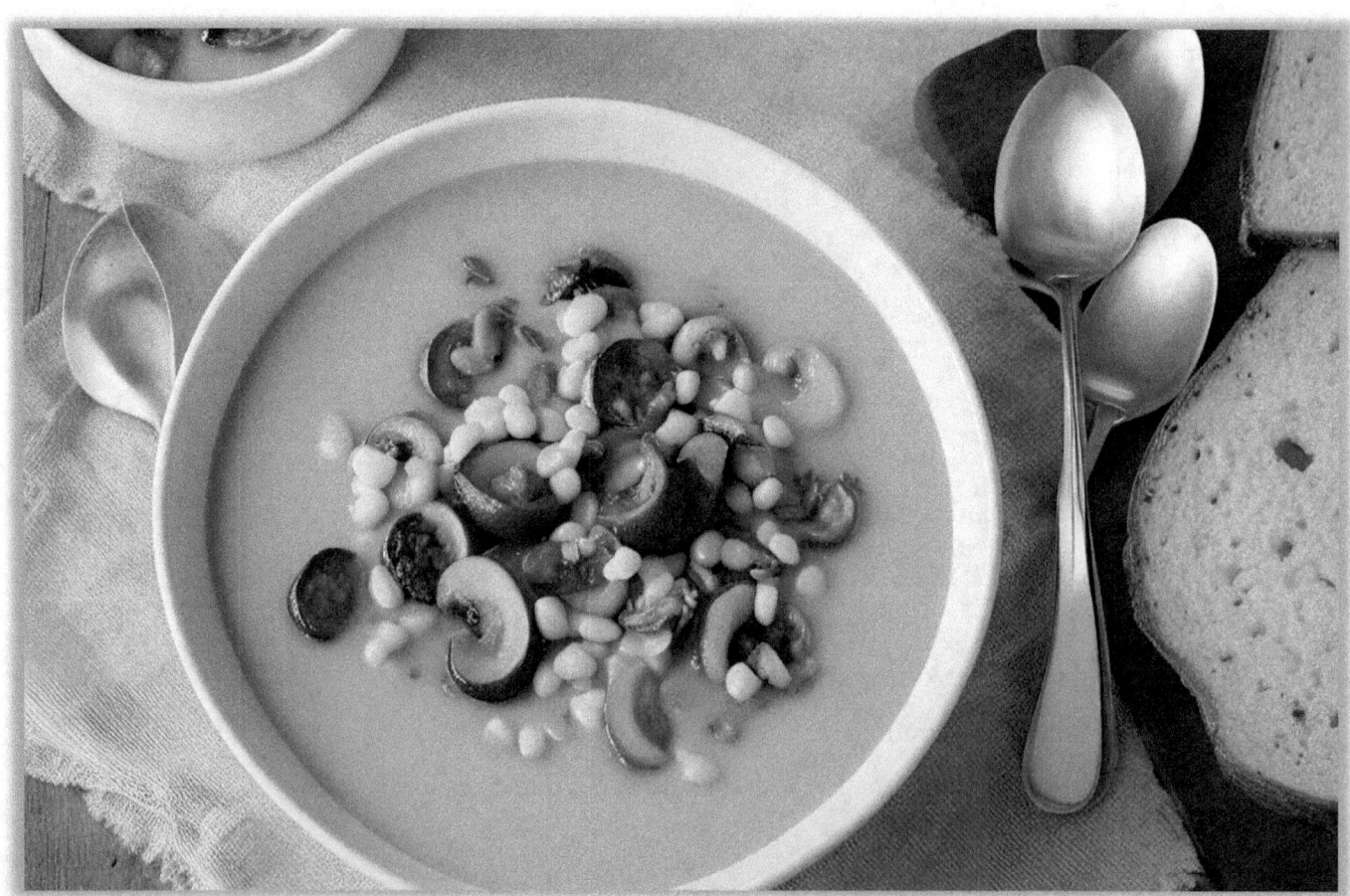

Curry-Ginger Vinaigrette

Liven up your CKD-friendly lunch salads with this flavorful and easy-to-make vinaigrette! Packed with warming spices and minimal potassium and phosphorus, it adds a delicious and kidney-friendly touch to your meal.

PREP TIME: 5 MINUTES | COOK TIME: NO COOK TIME | YIELDS: 1 SERVING

INGREDIENTS:

- 2 tablespoons olive oil
- 1 tablespoon lime juice
- 1 teaspoon low-sodium soy sauce
- ½ teaspoon grated ginger
- ¼ teaspoon curry powder
- Pinch of garlic powder
- Salt-free herb seasoning (to taste)

COOKING INSTRUCTIONS:

1. In a small bowl, whisk together olive oil, lime juice, soy sauce, ginger, curry powder, and garlic powder.
2. Season with salt-free herb seasoning to taste.
3. Serve immediately or store in an airtight container in the refrigerator for up to a week.

NUTRITIONAL INFORMATION: (APPROXIMATE VALUES PER SERVING)

Calories: 100

Phosphorus: 10mg

Protein: 0 grams

Sodium: 30mg (depending on seasoning)

Potassium: 20mg (depending on soy sauce)

TIPS FOR MODIFICATION:

- Choose low-sodium soy sauce: opt for a low-sodium soy sauce to control sodium intake.
- Potassium control: You can substitute tamari for soy sauce, if allowed in your diet. Tamari is a naturally gluten-free soy sauce that is often lower in potassium.

Beet Salad with Candied

This recipe uses modifications to minimize protein content while incorporating candied or spiced pecans for a satisfying and flavorful lunch option for those on a CKD diet.

PREP TIME: 10 MINUTES (DEPENDING ON BEET PREPARATION) | COOK TIME: ROASTING TIME FOR BEETS (VARIABLE) | YIELDS: 1 SERVING

INGREDIENTS:

- 1 cup chopped roasted beets (or pre-cooked canned beets, diced)
- ¼ cup chopped pecans (candied or spiced)
- 2 tablespoons crumbled goat cheese (optional)
- For the Vinaigrette:
- 1 tablespoon olive oil
- 1 tablespoon balsamic vinegar
- ½ teaspoon Dijon mustard (low-sodium option)
- Salt-free herb seasoning (to taste)

COOKING INSTRUCTIONS:

1. Prepare the beets: If using raw beets, roast them whole at 400°F (200°C) for 45-60 minutes, or until tender when pierced with a fork. Let cool, peel, and chop into bite-sized pieces. Alternatively, use pre-cooked and diced canned beets (ensure low-sodium options).
2. In a bowl, combine chopped beets and pecans.
3. For the Vinaigrette: In a separate small bowl, whisk together olive oil, balsamic vinegar, Dijon mustard, and salt-free herb seasoning to taste.
4. Drizzle the vinaigrette over the salad and toss to coat.
5. Top with crumbled goat cheese (optional) and serve immediately.

NUTRITIONAL INFORMATION: (APPROXIMATE VALUES PER SERVING)

Calories: 300   *Protein: 4 grams (from cheese and pecans)*

Potassium: 250mg (depending on beets)   *Sodium: 40mg (depending on seasoning)*

Phosphorus: 120mg (depending on cheese)

TIPS FOR MODIFICATION:

- For lower potassium: Choose pre-cooked and diced canned beets, and rinse them before using to remove some of the potassium content.
- Protein control: Skip the goat cheese or use a very minimal amount. You can substitute with a sprinkle of sunflower seeds for added texture.

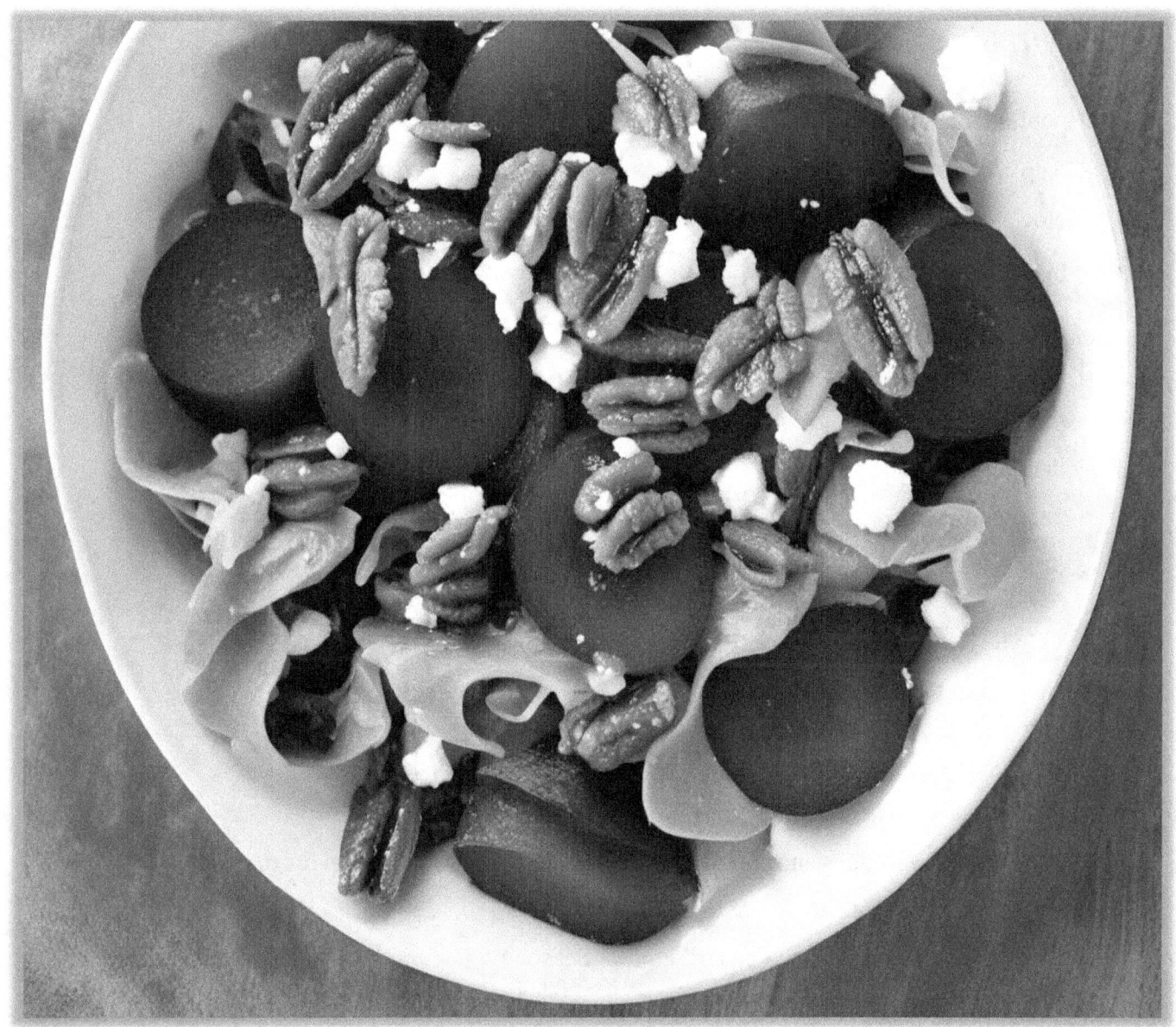

Smoky Corn and Chile Soup with CKD-Friendly Collard Greens

Enjoy a hearty and flavorful lunch that's kind to your kidneys! This recipe uses modifications to lower potassium and phosphorus while keeping the smoky depth and comforting textures of classic corn and Chile soup with collard greens.

PREP TIME: 10 MINUTES | COOK TIME: 25 MINUTES | YIELDS: 1 SERVING

INGREDIENTS:

- ½ tablespoon olive oil
- ½ cup chopped onion
- 1 clove garlic, minced
- 1 (4 oz) can diced green chiles (mild or fire-roasted, depending on preference)
- 1 cup low-sodium vegetable broth
- ½ cup frozen corn
- ½ cup chopped collard greens (rinsed and roughly chopped)
- ½ teaspoon ground cumin
- ¼ teaspoon smoked paprika
- Salt-free herb seasoning (to taste)

COOKING INSTRUCTIONS:

1. In a saucepan, heat olive oil over medium heat.
2. Add chopped onion and cook for 2-3 minutes, or until softened.
3. Add minced garlic and cook for an additional minute.
4. Stir in diced green chiles and cook for another minute, allowing the flavors to meld.
5. Pour in vegetable broth and bring to a simmer.
6. Add frozen corn and chopped collard greens. Season with cumin, smoked paprika, and a pinch of salt-free herb seasoning (optional).
7. Simmer for 15-20 minutes, or until the collard greens are tender and the corn is cooked through.

8. Adjust seasonings with additional salt-free herb seasoning to taste and serve hot.

NUTRITIONAL INFORMATION: (APPROXIMATE VALUES PER SERVING)

Calories: 200

Phosphorus: 80mg

Protein: 2 grams

Sodium: 40mg (depending on broth)

Potassium: 300mg (depending on collard greens)

TIPS FOR MODIFICATION:

- For lower potassium: Use a smaller amount of collard greens or choose a lower-potassium leafy green like spinach. You can also cook the greens separately and add them towards the end for less potassium leaching.
- Phosphorus control: opt for a pre-washed and chopped option for collard greens to minimize added sodium. You can also substitute with chopped cabbage for a similar texture (be mindful of portion size).

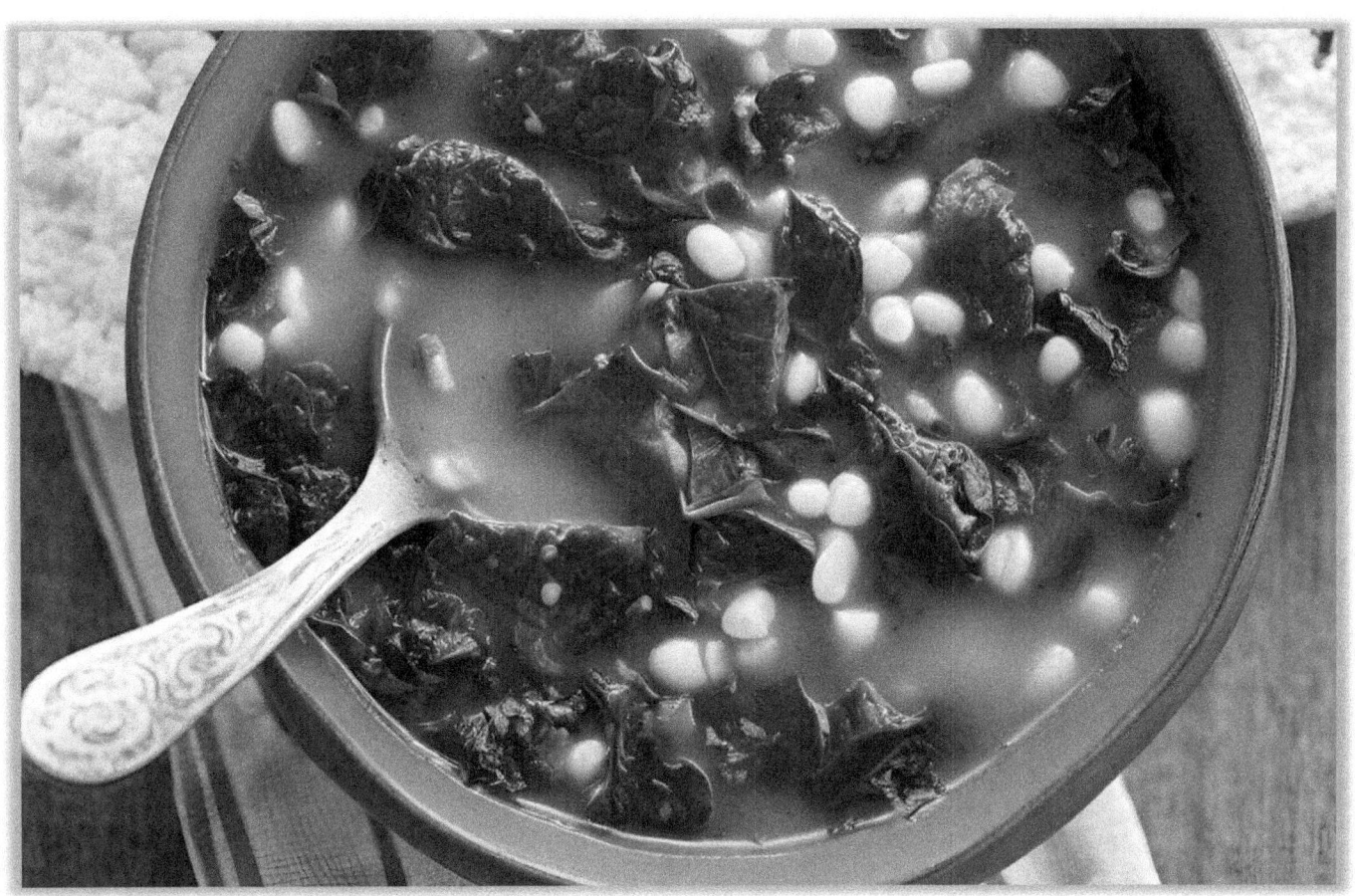

Tostada Salad

Give your taste buds a fiesta with this vibrant and kidney-friendly twist on the classic tostada salad! This recipe uses lower-potassium and lower-phosphorus ingredients to create a satisfying and flavorful lunch option for those on a CKD diet.

PREP TIME: 10 MINUTES | COOK TIME: NO COOK TIME | YIELDS: 1 SERVING

INGREDIENTS:

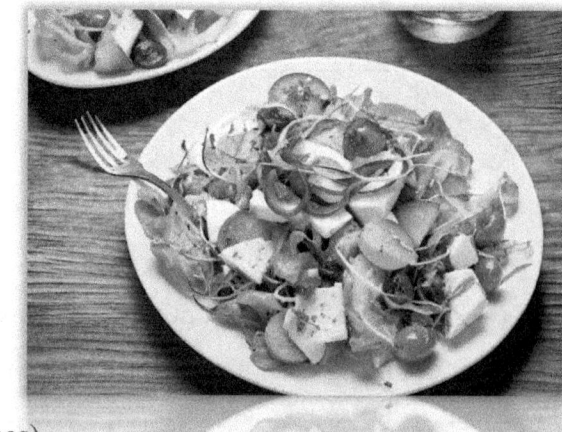

- ½ cup chopped romaine lettuce
- ¼ cup chopped bell pepper (any color)
- ¼ cup chopped black beans (rinsed and drained)
- ¼ cup chopped low-sodium salsa
- 2 tablespoons chopped fresh cilantro
- 1 tablespoon crumbled low-fat feta cheese (optional)
- 4 baked whole-wheat tortilla wedges (broken into pieces)

COOKING INSTRUCTIONS:

1. In a bowl, combine chopped romaine lettuce, bell pepper, black beans, salsa, and cilantro.
2. Top with crumbled feta cheese (optional) and baked whole-wheat tortilla wedges.

NUTRITIONAL INFORMATION: (APPROXIMATE VALUES PER SERVING)

Calories: 300

Phosphorus: 150mg (depending on cheese)

Protein: 8 grams (from beans and cheese)

Sodium: 100mg (depending on salsa)

Potassium: 300mg (depending on vegetables)

TIPS FOR MODIFICATION:

- For lower potassium: Choose green or yellow bell peppers over red peppers, as they tend to be lower in potassium. You can also rinse canned black beans before using them.
- Phosphorus control: Skip the feta cheese or use a very minimal amount. You can substitute with a sprinkle of sunflower seeds or chopped walnuts for added texture (be mindful of portion size).

Smoky Collard Greens

Enjoy the rich, smoky flavors of classic collard greens with a kidney-friendly twist! This recipe uses modifications to lower potassium and phosphorus while keeping the satisfying taste and texture, making it a perfect lunch option for those on a CKD diet.

PREP TIME: 10 MINUTES | COOK TIME: 20 MINUTES | YIELDS: 1 SERVING

INGREDIENTS:

- ½ tablespoon olive oil
- ½ cup chopped onion
- 1 clove garlic, minced
- 2 cups chopped collard greens (rinsed and roughly chopped)
- ½ cup low-sodium vegetable broth
- 1 tablespoon apple cider vinegar
- ¼ teaspoon smoked paprika
- Pinch of black pepper
- Salt-free herb seasoning (to taste)

COOKING INSTRUCTIONS:

1. In a large skillet, heat olive oil over medium heat.
2. Add chopped onion and cook for 2-3 minutes, or until softened.
3. Add minced garlic and cook for an additional minute.
4. Stir in chopped collard greens and cook for another 2-3 minutes, or until slightly wilted.
5. Pour in vegetable broth and apple cider vinegar. Season with smoked paprika, black pepper, and a pinch of salt-free herb seasoning (optional).
6. Bring to a simmer, cover, and cook for 15-20 minutes, or until the collard greens are tender and flavorful.
7. Adjust seasonings with additional salt-free herb seasoning to taste and serve hot.

NUTRITIONAL INFORMATION: (APPROXIMATE VALUES PER SERVING)

Calories: 150

Phosphorus: 80mg

Protein: 2 grams

Sodium: 40mg (depending on broth)

Potassium: 350mg (depending on collard greens)

TIPS FOR MODIFICATION:

- For lower potassium: Use a smaller amount of collard greens or choose a lower-potassium leafy green like spinach. You can also cook the greens separately and add them towards the end for less potassium leaching.
- Phosphorus control: opt for a pre-washed and chopped option for collard greens to minimize added sodium. You can also substitute with chopped cabbage for a similar texture (be mindful of portion size).

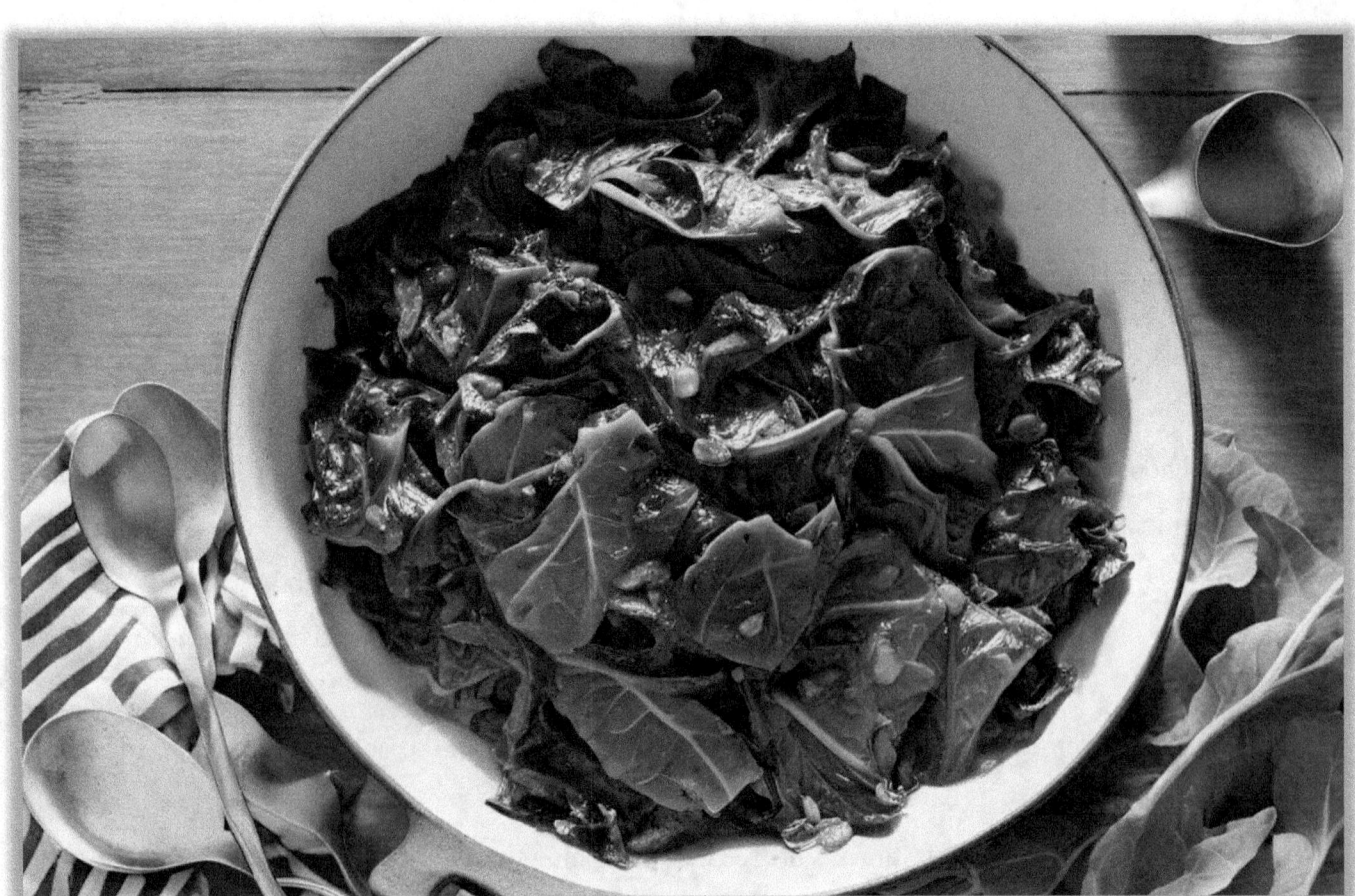

DINNER RECIPES

Welcome to Our Kidney-Friendly Dinner Recipes

Dinner is the moment when we can finally relax and enjoy a delicious meal without the chaos of the day. And guess what? Eating healthy doesn't mean saying goodbye to flavor. In fact, our dinner recipes will make your taste buds dance with joy! Tailored specifically for Stage 3 kidney disease, these dishes are low in protein, potassium, sodium, and phosphorus – but high in yum.

What to Expect

1. Flavorful and Hearty Dishes: Get ready for some seriously hearty meals like Portobello Steaks with Twice-Cooked Mashed Potatoes and Balsamic Arugula, and Mushroom Bourguignon. These dishes are so flavorful, even your non-kidney-disease friends will be begging for a bite.
2. Fresh and Light Options: Lighten things up with Pineapple and Vegetable Kebabs, Watermelon Gazpacho, and Charred Romaine with Caesar Dressing. Perfect for those nights when you want something refreshing and guilt-free.
3. Bold and Spicy Flavors: Bring on the zest with Mexican Street Corn Salad, Vegetable Fajitas, and Jackfruit "Carnitas" Tacos. Your taste buds will be throwing a fiesta!
4. Innovative and Creative Recipes: Try out unique dishes like Italian Pesto Zucchini Noodles, Ginger-Garlic Vegetable Ramen Bowls, and Tortilla Soup. Who knew kidney-friendly could be so inventive?
5. Versatile Sides and Sauces: Boost your meals with sides and sauces like Vinegar Slaw, Louisiana Remoulade, and No-Sodium Umami Sauce. They're like the secret weapons of your dinner plate.
6. Nutritious and Satisfying Salads: Dive into salads like Main Dish Salad and Pepper Salad, which are so filling they can be a meal on their own or a satisfying side.

Here's to you, brave culinary explorer! You have made it this far, navigating the wild world of kidney-friendly cooking with determination. Keep going, and remember: eating well is the best way to show your kidneys some love. Enjoy your dinners, and don't forget to have fun along the way!

Mexican Street Corn Salad (Esquites)

Enjoy the bold flavors of Mexico with a kidney-friendly twist! This vibrant Esquites recipe uses modifications to lower phosphorus and potassium while keeping the fresh and satisfying taste of grilled corn and creamy dressing. Perfect for a light and flavorful lunch on a CKD diet.

PREP TIME: 15 MINUTES | COOK TIME: 10 MINUTES (GRILLING) | YIELDS: 1 SERVING

INGREDIENTS:

- 1 ear fresh corn, shucked and kernels removed (about ½ cup)
- ½ tablespoon olive oil
- ¼ cup chopped red onion
- ¼ cup chopped fresh cilantro
- 2 tablespoons crumbled Cotija cheese (potassium watch!) OR crumbled feta cheese
- 1 tablespoon low-fat mayonnaise
- 1 tablespoon lime juice
- Chili powder (to taste)
- Salt-free herb seasoning (to taste)

COOKING INSTRUCTIONS:

1. Heat olive oil in a grill pan or skillet over medium heat.
2. Add corn kernels and cook for 5-7 minutes, stirring occasionally, until lightly charred.
3. While corn cooks, combine chopped red onion, cilantro, and chosen cheese (Cotija or feta) in a bowl.
4. In a separate small bowl, whisk together mayonnaise, lime juice, chili powder, and salt-free herb seasoning to taste.
5. Once corn is cooked, add it to the bowl with the vegetables and cheese.
6. Pour the dressing over the salad and toss to coat.
7. Serve immediately and enjoy!

NUTRITIONAL INFORMATION: (APPROXIMATE VALUES PER SERVING)

Calories: 250

Phosphorus: 150mg (depending on cheese)

Protein: 4 grams (from cheese)

Sodium: 40mg (depending on seasoning)

Potassium: 250mg (depending on cheese)

TIPS FOR MODIFICATION:

- Cheese Choice: opt for feta cheese instead of Cotija cheese, as it's generally lower in potassium.
- Portion Control: Limit the amount of cheese used due to its phosphorus content.

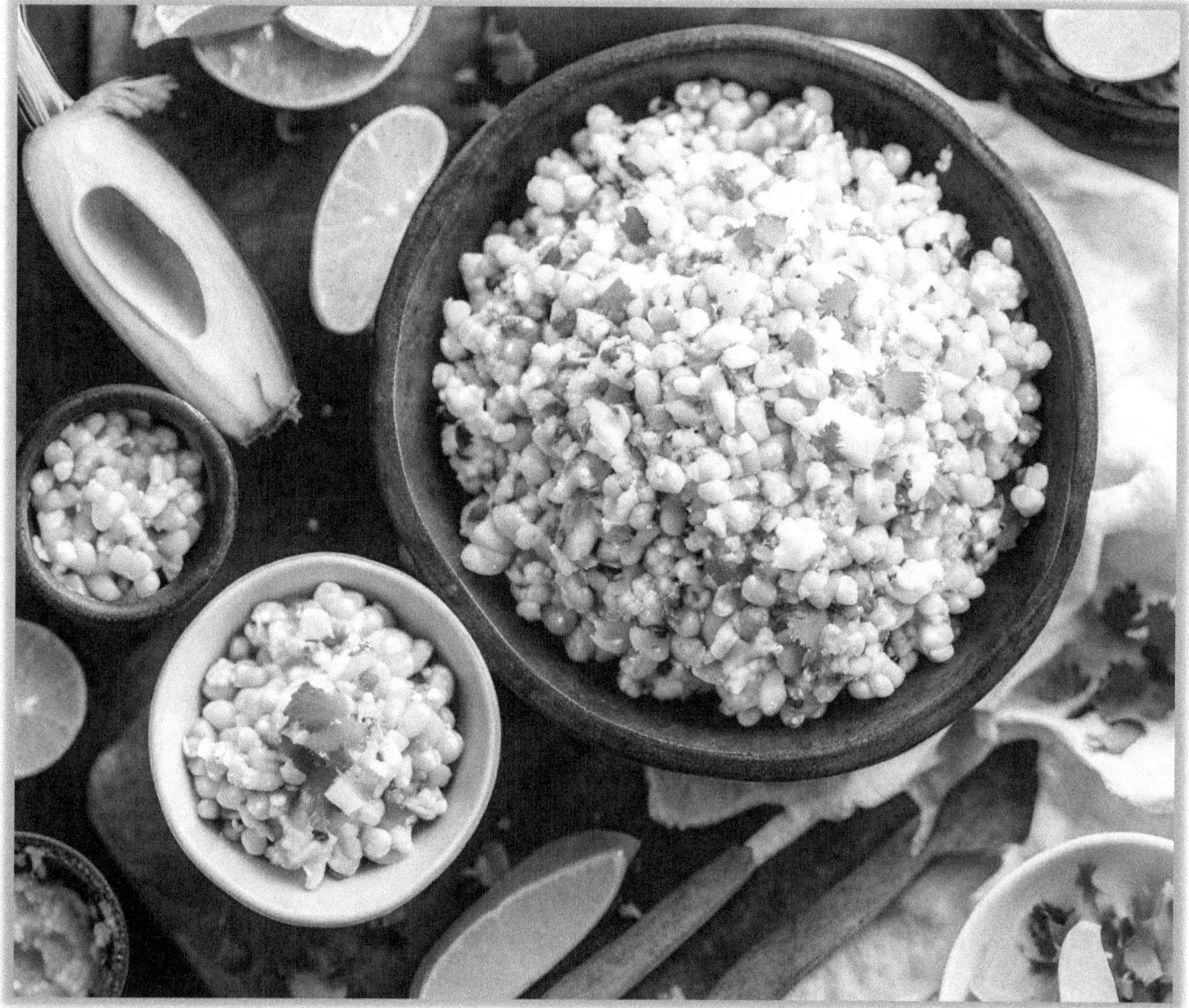

Veggie Fajitas

Sizzle up a fiesta of flavors with these easy and kidney-friendly veggie fajitas! This recipe uses a colorful mix of vegetables and swaps traditional high-potassium options for a satisfying and flavorful dinner perfect for a CKD diet.

PREP TIME: 15 MINUTES | COOK TIME: 15-20 MINUTES | YIELDS: 1 SERVING

INGREDIENTS:

- 1 tablespoon olive oil
- ½ cup chopped onion
- 1 bell pepper (any color), sliced
- ½ cup sliced zucchini
- ½ cup chopped mushrooms (optional)
- ½ cup chopped low-sodium salsa (or Pico de Gallo)
- 1 tablespoon lime juice
- 1 teaspoon chili powder
- ¼ teaspoon ground cumin
- Pinch of smoked paprika (optional)
- Salt-free herb seasoning (to taste)
- 2 low-carb tortillas (whole wheat, corn, etc.)

COOKING INSTRUCTIONS:

1. Heat olive oil in a large skillet or grill pan over medium-high heat.
2. Add chopped onion and cook for 3-4 minutes, or until softened.
3. Add bell pepper slices, zucchini slices, and mushrooms (if using) and cook for an additional 5-7 minutes, or until tender-crisp.
4. While the vegetables cook, in a small bowl, combine salsa, lime juice, chili powder, cumin, smoked paprika (optional), and salt-free herb seasoning to taste.
5. Warm your tortillas according to package instructions.

6. Once the vegetables are cooked, spoon them into the warmed tortillas and top with your prepared salsa mixture.

NUTRITIONAL INFORMATION: (APPROXIMATE VALUES PER SERVING)

Calories: 350

Phosphorus: 100mg

Protein: 2 grams

Sodium: 150mg (depending on salsa)

Potassium: 400mg (depending on vegetables)

TIPS FOR MODIFICATION:

- Potassium Control: Choose green or yellow bell peppers over red peppers, as they tend to be lower in potassium. You can also rinse canned vegetables before using them.
- Low-Carb Options: Select low-carb tortillas or use lettuce wraps as an alternative for a more kidney-friendly option.

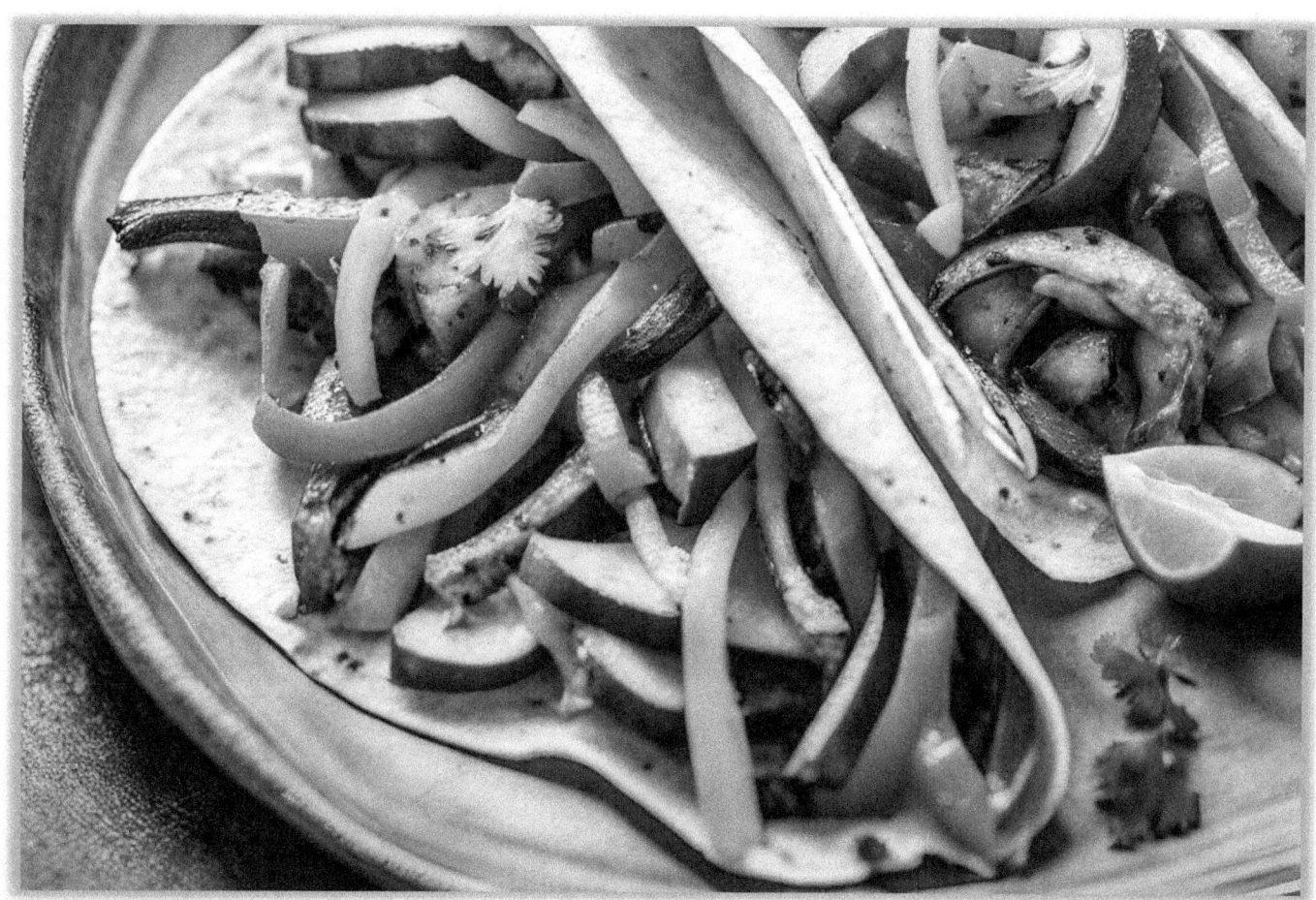

Portobello Steaks with Mashed Cauliflower and Balsamic Arugula

Portobello mushroom steaks are marinated and grilled to perfection, served with a creamy mashed cauliflower option and a refreshing balsamic arugula salad.

PREP TIME: 15 MINUTES | COOK TIME: 20-25 MINUTES | YIELDS: 1 SERVING

INGREDIENTS:

- 1 large portobello mushroom cap

For the Marinade:

- 1 tablespoon olive oil
- 1 tablespoon balsamic vinegar
- 1 teaspoon low-sodium soy sauce
- ½ teaspoon dried thyme
- Pinch of garlic powder
- Black pepper (to taste)

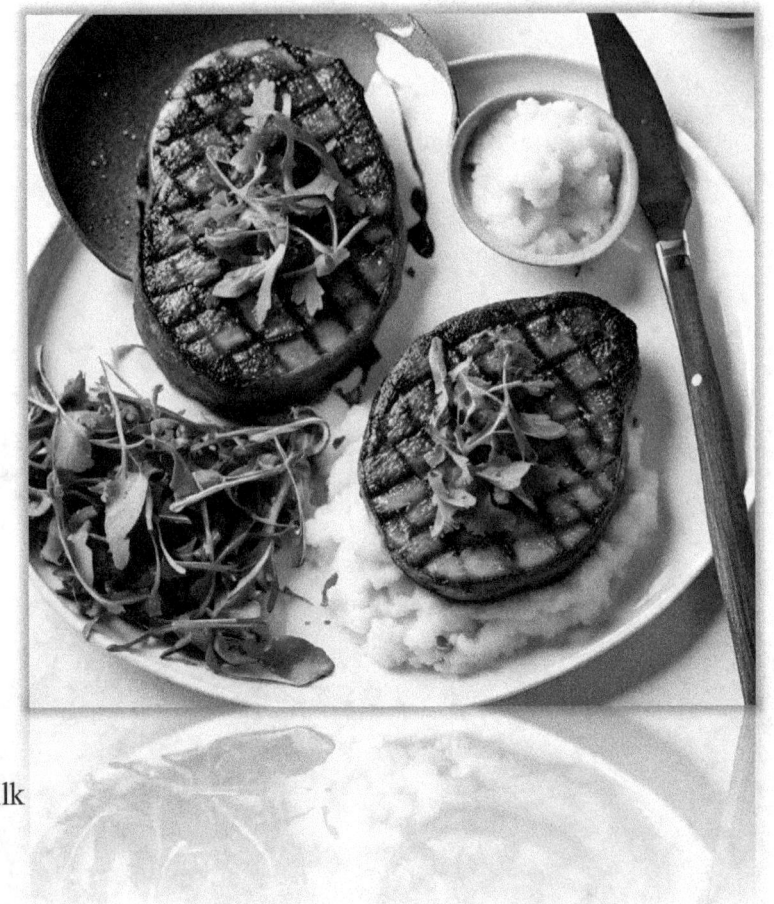

For the Mashed Cauliflower:

- 1 cup chopped cauliflower florets
- 2 tablespoons unsweetened almond milk
- 1 tablespoon butter
- Salt-free herb seasoning (to taste)

Balsamic Arugula Salad:

- ½ cup arugula
- 1 tablespoon balsamic vinegar
- ½ tablespoon olive oil

- Salt-free herb seasoning (to taste)

COOKING INSTRUCTIONS:

1. Marinate the portobello: In a shallow dish, whisk together olive oil, balsamic vinegar, soy sauce, thyme, garlic powder, and black pepper. Add the portobello mushroom cap (gills facing down) and marinate for 15 minutes.
2. Prepare the mashed cauliflower: In a small saucepan, steam or boil cauliflower florets until tender. Drain any excess water.
3. In the same saucepan, mash the cauliflower florets with almond milk and butter. Season with salt-free herb seasoning to taste. Set aside.
4. Cook the portobello steak: Heat a grill pan or skillet over medium-high heat. Remove the portobello mushroom cap from the marinade and cook for 5-7 minutes per side, or until tender and slightly charred.
5. Assemble the dish: In a bowl, toss arugula with balsamic vinegar, olive oil, and salt-free herb seasoning to taste.
6. Plate the mashed cauliflower, top with the cooked portobello steak, and serve with the balsamic arugula salad on the side.

NUTRITIONAL INFORMATION: (APPROXIMATE VALUES PER SERVING)

Calories: 400

Protein: 8 grams (from portobello mushroom)

Potassium: 350mg (depending on vegetables)

Phosphorus: 200mg (depending on cauliflower)

Sodium: 100mg (depending on seasoning)

TIPS FOR MODIFICATION:

- For lower phosphorus: You can substitute mashed zucchini or turnips for the mashed cauliflower.
- Potassium control: Rinse the portobello mushroom cap before marinating to remove some of the potassium content. opt for a light balsamic glaze instead of the balsamic arugula salad if potassium is a major concern.

Italian Pesto Zucchini Noodles

This recipe uses zucchini noodles instead of traditional pasta, tossed in a delicious pesto and packed with minimal phosphorus and potassium. Perfect for a satisfying and kidney-friendly meal on a CKD diet.

PREP TIME: 10 MINUTES | COOK TIME: 5 MINUTES (DEPENDING ON COOKING METHOD FOR ZUCCHINI NOODLES) | YIELDS: 1 SERVING

INGREDIENTS:

- 2 small zucchinis, spiralized into noodles (or use a julienne peeler)
- ½ cup prepared pesto (store-bought or homemade)
- Cherry tomatoes (optional)
- Fresh basil leaves (for garnish, optional)
- Salt-free herb seasoning (to taste)

COOKING INSTRUCTIONS:

1. Prepare the zucchini noodles: Using a spiralizer or julienne peeler, create zucchini noodles from the zucchini. You can also substitute pre-spiralized zucchini noodles if desired.
2. There are two options for cooking the zucchini noodles:
3. Sautéing: Heat a pan with a drizzle of olive oil over medium heat. Add the zucchini noodles and cook for 2-3 minutes, or until tender-crisp (not mushy).
4. Microwaving: Place the zucchini noodles in a microwave-safe bowl with a splash of water. Cover and microwave on high for 1-2 minutes, or until tender-crisp. Drain any excess water.
5. In a large bowl, toss the cooked zucchini noodles with your desired amount of pesto.
6. Plate the pesto zucchini noodles and garnish with cherry tomatoes and fresh basil leaves (optional). Season with a sprinkle of salt-free herb seasoning to taste.

NUTRITIONAL INFORMATION: (APPROXIMATE VALUES PER SERVING)

Calories: 300 (depending on pesto)

Potassium: 300mg (depending on vegetables)

Protein: 4 grams (from pesto)

Phosphorus: 80mg

Sodium: 100mg (depending on pesto)

TIPS FOR MODIFICATION:

- Choose Low-Potassium Pesto: opt for a store-bought pesto labeled "low-sodium" or "sodium-free" as they tend to be lower in potassium as well.
- Portion Control: Be mindful of the amount of pesto used, as it can vary in phosphorus content depending on the recipe.

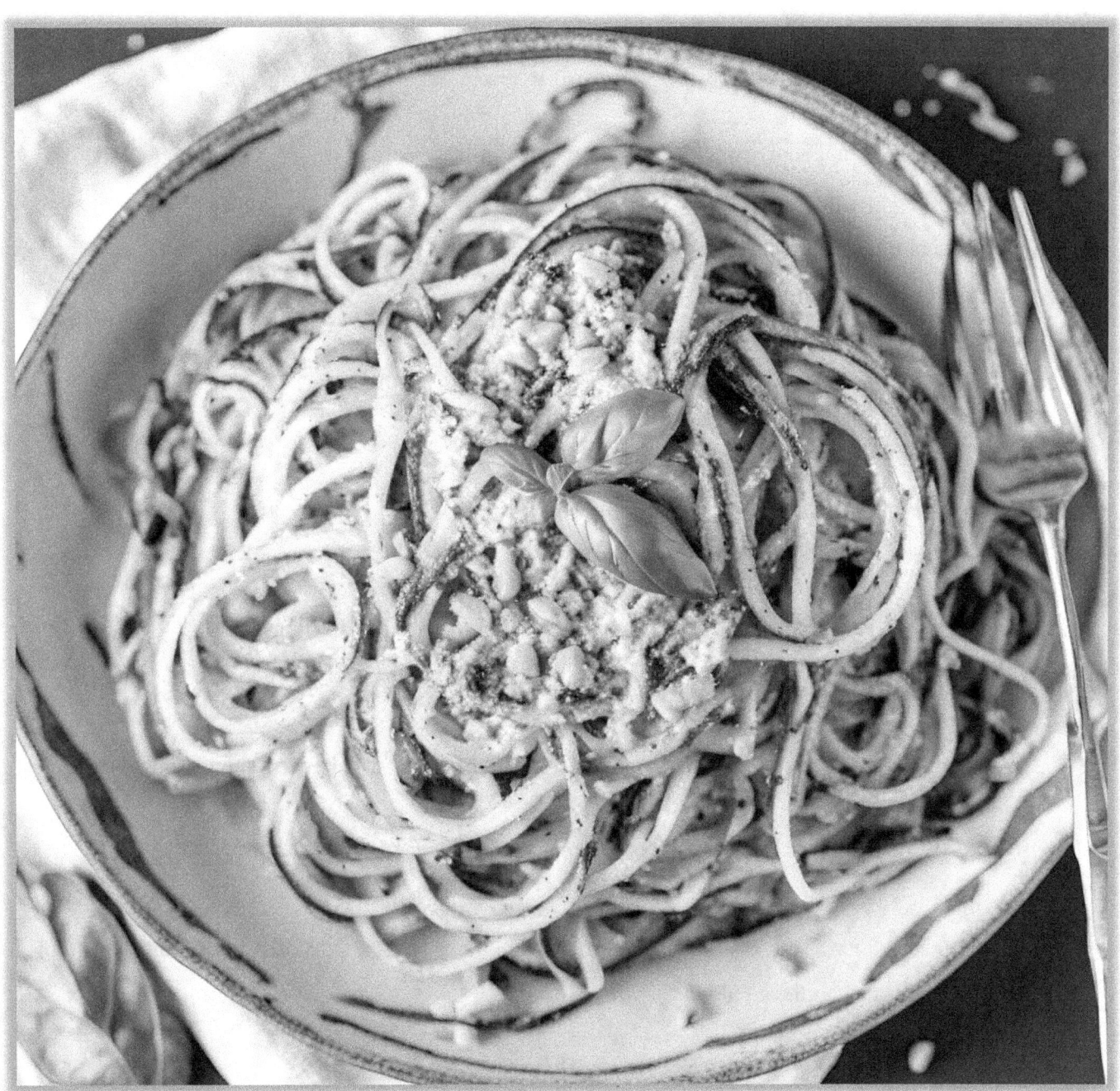

Pineapple and Veggie Kebabs

These vibrant pineapple and veggie kebabs are perfect for a fun and flavorful dinner on a CKD diet! This recipe uses lower-potassium vegetables and pineapple chunks, skewered and grilled or baked for a satisfying and healthy meal.

PREP TIME: 10 MINUTES | COOK TIME: 10-15 MINUTES (GRILLING) OR 20-25 MINUTES (BAKING) | YIELDS: 1 SERVING

INGREDIENTS:

- 1/4 cup chopped pineapple chunks (fresh or canned in water, drained)
- ¼ cup bell pepper (any color), cut into chunks
- ¼ cup zucchini, cut into chunks
- ¼ cup red onion, cut into wedges
- 1 tablespoon olive oil
- Salt-free herb seasoning (to taste)
- Skewers (wooden or metal)

COOKING INSTRUCTIONS:

1. Preheat grill or oven to medium heat (around 400°F).
2. Soak wooden skewers in water for 10 minutes if using (to prevent burning).
3. Thread pineapple chunks, bell pepper pieces, zucchini chunks, and red onion wedges alternately onto skewers.
4. In a small bowl, toss olive oil with salt-free herb seasoning to taste. Brush the kabobs with the oil mixture.
5. Grilling method: Grill the kabobs for 8-10 minutes per side, or until vegetables are tender-crisp and pineapple is slightly charred.
6. Baking method: Place the kabobs on a baking sheet and bake for 20-25 minutes, or until vegetables are tender and pineapple is golden brown.
7. Serve immediately and enjoy!

NUTRITIONAL INFORMATION: (APPROXIMATE VALUES PER SERVING)

Calories: 200

Phosphorus: 50mg

Protein: 1 gram

Sodium: 30mg (depending on seasoning)

Potassium: 200mg (depending on vegetables)

TIPS FOR MODIFICATION:

- Potassium control: Choose green or yellow bell peppers over red peppers, as they tend to be lower in potassium. You can also rinse canned pineapple chunks before using them to remove some potassium content.
- Vegetable Selection: If potassium is a major concern, substitute lower-potassium vegetables like mushrooms or cherry tomatoes for the bell pepper or onion.

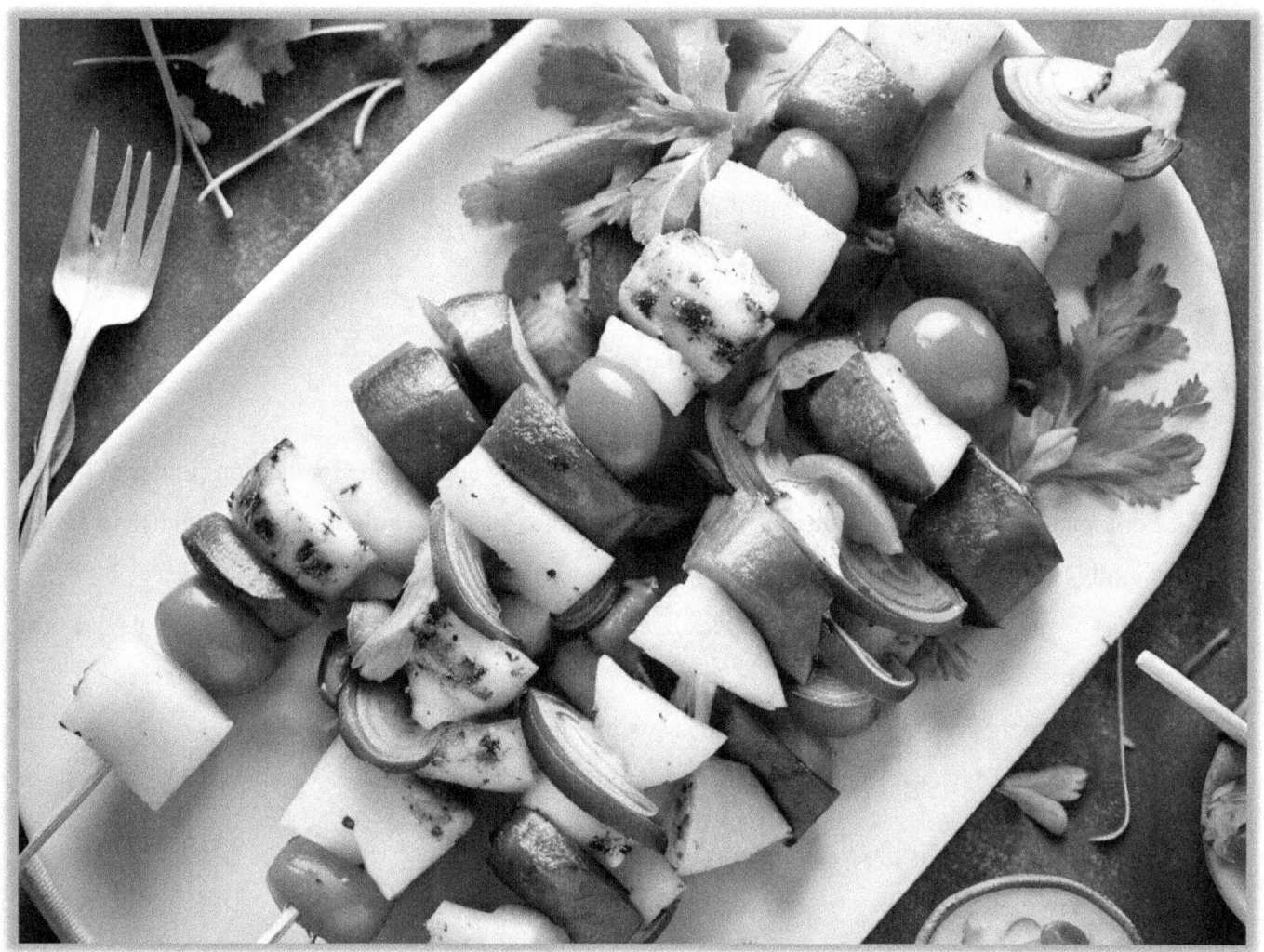

Refreshing Vinegar Slaw

Cool down your dinner plate with this tangy and crunchy vinegar slaw! This side dish is perfect for those on a CKD diet, featuring shredded vegetables with a flavorful vinaigrette dressing that's lower in phosphorus and potassium.

PREP TIME: 10 MINUTES | COOK TIME: NO COOK TIME (MARINATING RECOMMENDED) | YIELDS: 1 SERVING

INGREDIENTS:

- 2 cups shredded cabbage (green or purple)
- ¼ cup grated carrots
- 1 tablespoon chopped red onion (optional)
- For the Vinaigrette:
- 2 tablespoons olive oil
- 2 tablespoons white vinegar
- 1 teaspoon Dijon mustard (low-sodium option)
- ½ teaspoon dried dill
- Salt-free herb seasoning (to taste)

COOKING INSTRUCTIONS:

1. In a large bowl, combine shredded cabbage, grated carrots, and chopped red onion (if using).
2. For a more flavorful slaw (optional): Let the vegetables sit in the bowl for 15-20 minutes to soften slightly.
3. In a separate small bowl, whisk together olive oil, white vinegar, Dijon mustard, dried dill, and salt-free herb seasoning to taste.
4. Pour the vinaigrette dressing over the coleslaw mix and toss to coat evenly.
5. Serve immediately or refrigerate for up to 30 minutes for chilled slaw.

NUTRITIONAL INFORMATION: (APPROXIMATE VALUES PER SERVING)

Calories: 150   *Protein: 1 gram*

Potassium: 250mg (depending on vegetables)   *Sodium: 30mg (depending on seasoning)*

Phosphorus: 40mg

TIPS FOR MODIFICATION:

- Potassium control: opt for green cabbage over purple cabbage, as it's generally lower in potassium. You can also rinse the shredded cabbage before using to remove some potassium content.
- Reduce Phosphorus: Skip the red onion or use a minimal amount, as it can be higher in phosphorus. Chopped celery can be a good lower-phosphorus substitute.

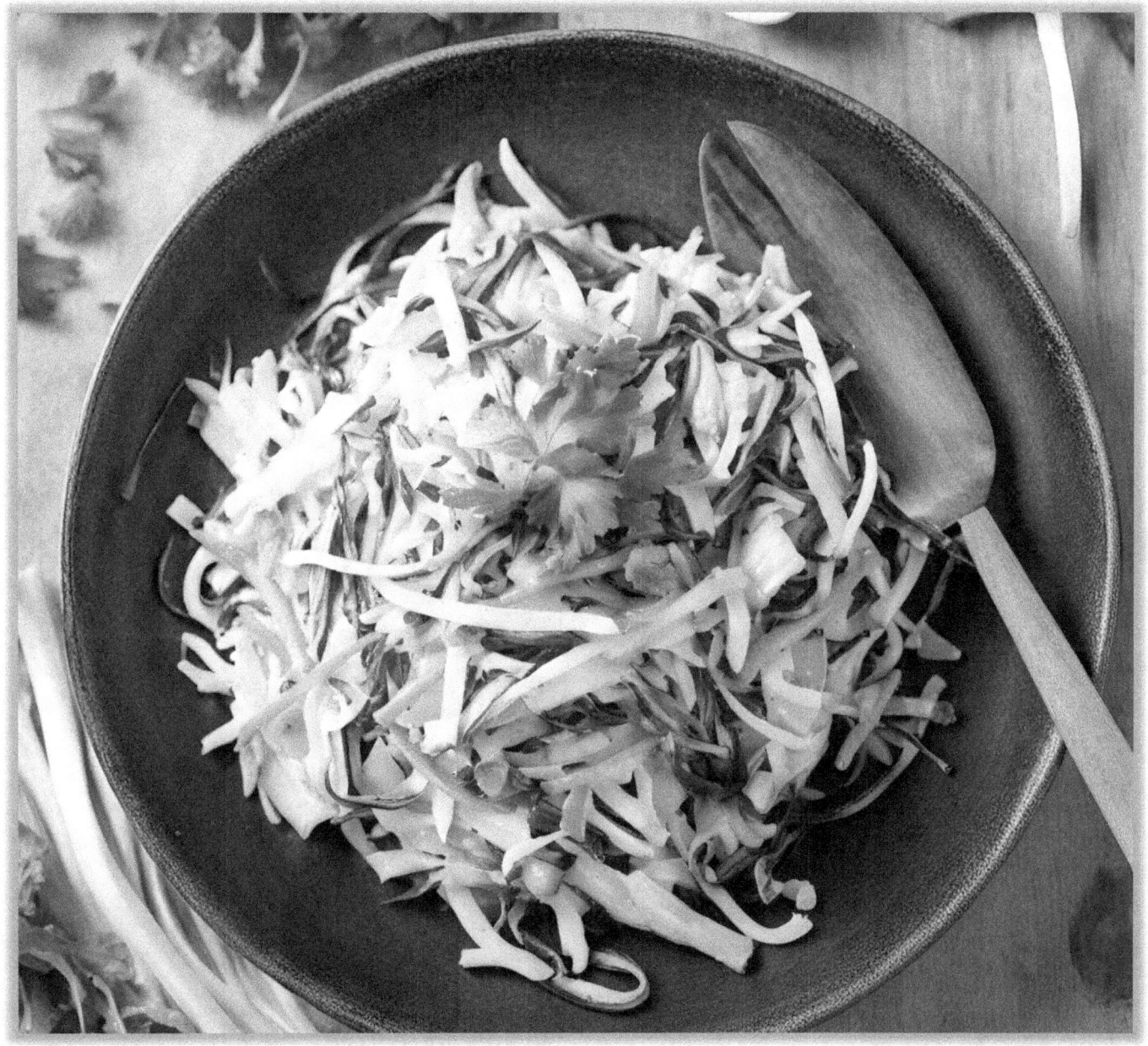

Louisiana Remoulade

Add a creamy and flavorful kick to your dinner with this Louisiana Remoulade recipe! This version is adapted for a CKD diet, using modifications to lower phosphorus and potassium while keeping the classic taste and texture. Perfect for dipping or dressing various dishes.

PREP TIME: 10 MINUTES | COOK TIME: NO COOK TIME | YIELDS: 1 SERVING

INGREDIENTS:

- ⅔ cup mayonnaise (low-fat or light option)
- 1 tablespoon whole grain mustard
- 1 tablespoon prepared horseradish (low-sodium option)
- 1 tablespoon chopped fresh parsley
- 1 tablespoon chopped green onions
- 1 teaspoon dried chives
- ½ teaspoon paprika
- Pinch of cayenne pepper (optional)
- Salt-free herb seasoning (to taste)

COOKING INSTRUCTIONS:

1. In a small bowl, whisk together mayonnaise, mustard, horseradish, parsley, green onions, chives, paprika, and cayenne pepper (if using).
2. Season with salt-free herb seasoning to taste.
3. Cover and refrigerate for at least 30 minutes to allow flavors to meld.

NUTRITIONAL INFORMATION: (APPROXIMATE VALUES PER SERVING)

Calories: 200

Potassium: 150mg (depending on ingredients)

Protein: 2 grams

Phosphorus: 100mg (depending on ingredients)

Sodium: 50mg (depending on ingredients)

TIPS FOR MODIFICATION:

- Lower Potassium: Choose low-potassium herbs like dill or chives instead of parsley. You can also rinse fresh herbs before using them.
- Phosphorus Management: opt for a light mayonnaise option or use less mayonnaise overall. Consider substituting a small amount of plain, unsweetened Greek yogurt for some of the mayonnaise for added protein.

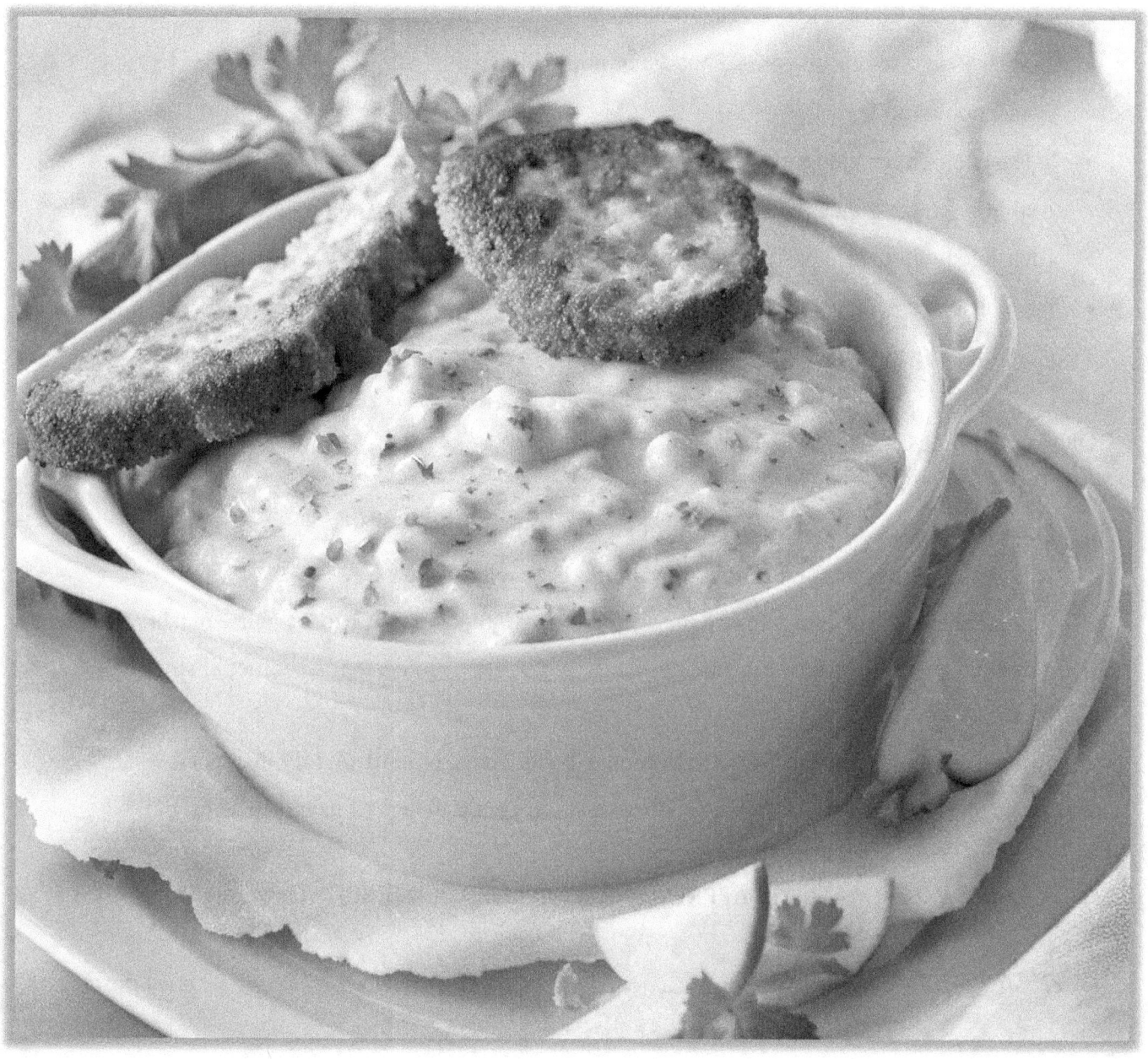

No-Sodium Uwami Sauce

This recipe for No-Sodium Uwami Sauce is perfect for a CKD-friendly dinner, using ingredients strategically chosen to lower sodium while maintaining a delicious taste profile.

PREP TIME: 5 MINUTES | COOK TIME: 10 MINUTES | YIELDS: 1 SERVING

INGREDIENTS:

- 1 cup vegetable broth (low-sodium option)
- 1 tablespoon dried mushrooms (shiitake or portobello)
- 1 teaspoon minced garlic
- ½ teaspoon grated ginger
- 1 tablespoon soy sauce (potassium watch!) - low-sodium tamari recommended
- 1 teaspoon white miso paste (or use more low-sodium soy sauce)
- Pinch of black pepper
- Pinch of red pepper flakes (optional)

COOKING INSTRUCTIONS:

1. In a small saucepan, heat vegetable broth over medium heat.
2. Add dried mushrooms and simmer for 5 minutes to release their flavor.
3. Strain the broth to remove mushroom pieces (or leave them in for a more intense mushroom flavor).
4. Add minced garlic, grated ginger, soy sauce, and white miso paste (or additional soy sauce) to the broth.
5. Bring to a simmer and cook for an additional 2-3 minutes, or until slightly thickened.
6. Remove from heat and stir in black pepper and red pepper flakes (if using) to taste.

NUTRITIONAL INFORMATION: (APPROXIMATE VALUES PER SERVING)

Calories: 50 *Protein: 2 grams (depending on miso paste)*

Potassium: 200mg (depending on ingredients)   *Sodium: 80mg (depending on soy sauce)*

Phosphorus: 50mg (depending on ingredients)

TIPS FOR MODIFICATION:

- Potassium Control: Use a low-sodium tamari instead of soy sauce, as it's typically lower in potassium. Consider using a smaller amount or omitting entirely if potassium is a major concern.
- Phosphorus Management: opt for white miso paste over other miso varieties, as it's generally lower in phosphorus. You can also skip the miso paste altogether for a purely soy sauce-based uwami sauce.

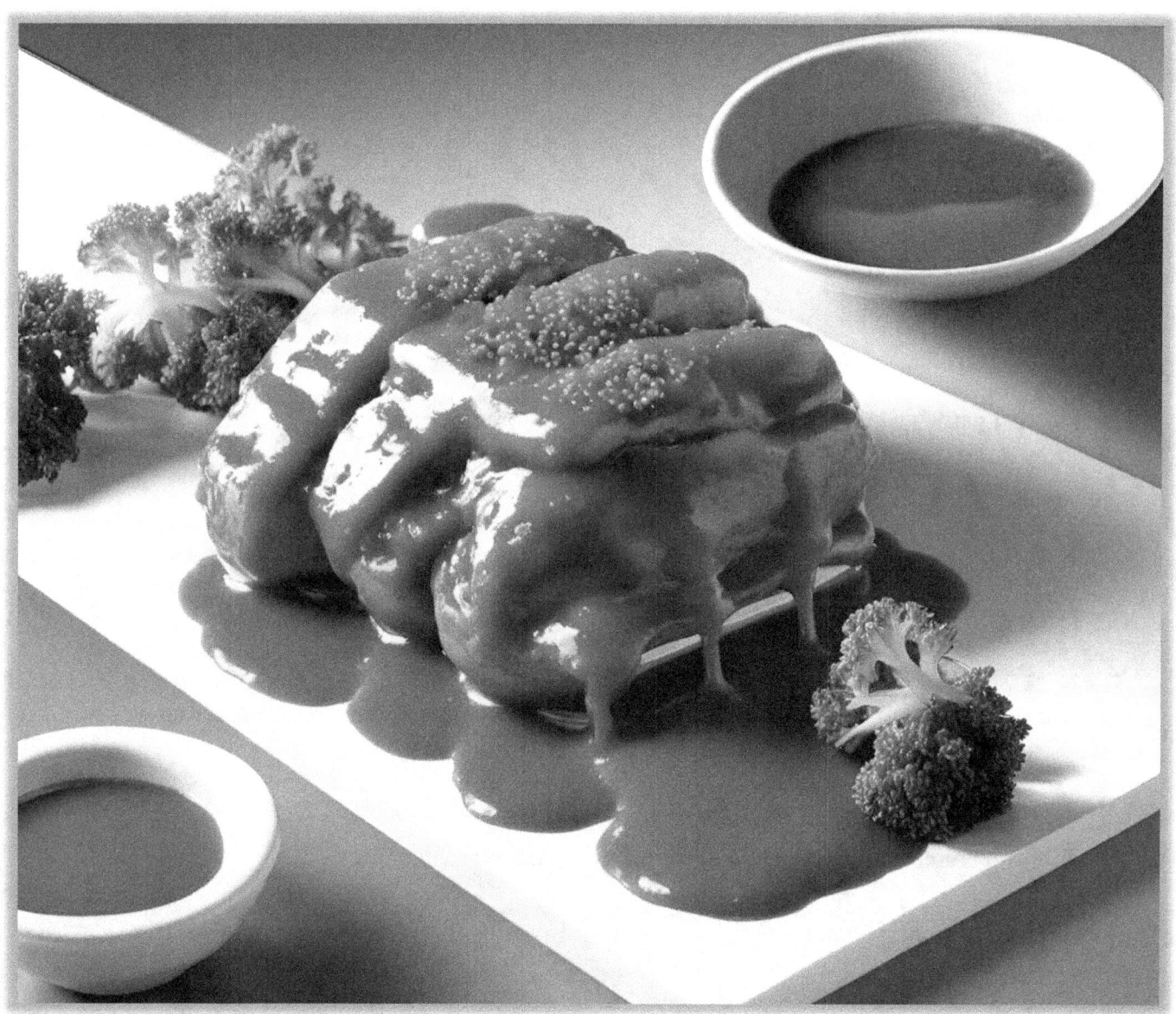

Summery Pepper Salad

Cool off your dinner plate with this vibrant and flavorful pepper salad! This side dish is perfect for a CKD diet, featuring a medley of colorful bell peppers with a simple and light dressing.

PREP TIME: 10 MINUTES | COOK TIME: NO COOK TIME (MARINATING RECOMMENDED) | YIELDS: 1 SERVING

INGREDIENTS:

- 1 bell pepper (any color, or a mix) thinly sliced
- ¼ cup cucumber, thinly sliced
- 2 cherry tomatoes, halved
- 1 tablespoon crumbled feta cheese (potassium watch!) OR crumbled low-fat ricotta cheese

For the Dressing:

- 1 tablespoon olive oil
- 1 tablespoon lemon juice
- ½ teaspoon dried oregano
- Pinch of garlic powder
- Salt-free herb seasoning (to taste)

COOKING INSTRUCTIONS:

1. In a medium bowl, combine sliced bell pepper, cucumber, and cherry tomatoes.
2. For extra flavor (optional): Let the vegetables sit in the bowl for 15-20 minutes to marinate slightly.
3. In a separate small bowl, whisk together olive oil, lemon juice, dried oregano, garlic powder, and salt-free herb seasoning to taste.
4. Pour the dressing over the salad and toss to coat evenly.
5. Top with crumbled feta cheese (or ricotta cheese) and serve immediately.

Nutritional Information: (approximate values per serving)

Calories: 150   *Protein: 2 grams (from cheese)*

Potassium: 300mg (depending on vegetables and cheese)

Sodium: 40mg (depending on seasoning and cheese)

Phosphorus: 100mg (depending on cheese)

TIPS FOR MODIFICATION:

- Cheese Choice: opt for low-fat ricotta cheese instead of feta cheese, as it's generally lower in potassium and phosphorus. You can also skip the cheese altogether for a vegan option.
- Potassium Control: Choose green or yellow bell peppers over red peppers, as they tend to be lower in potassium. You can also rinse the bell peppers before slicing to remove some potassium content.

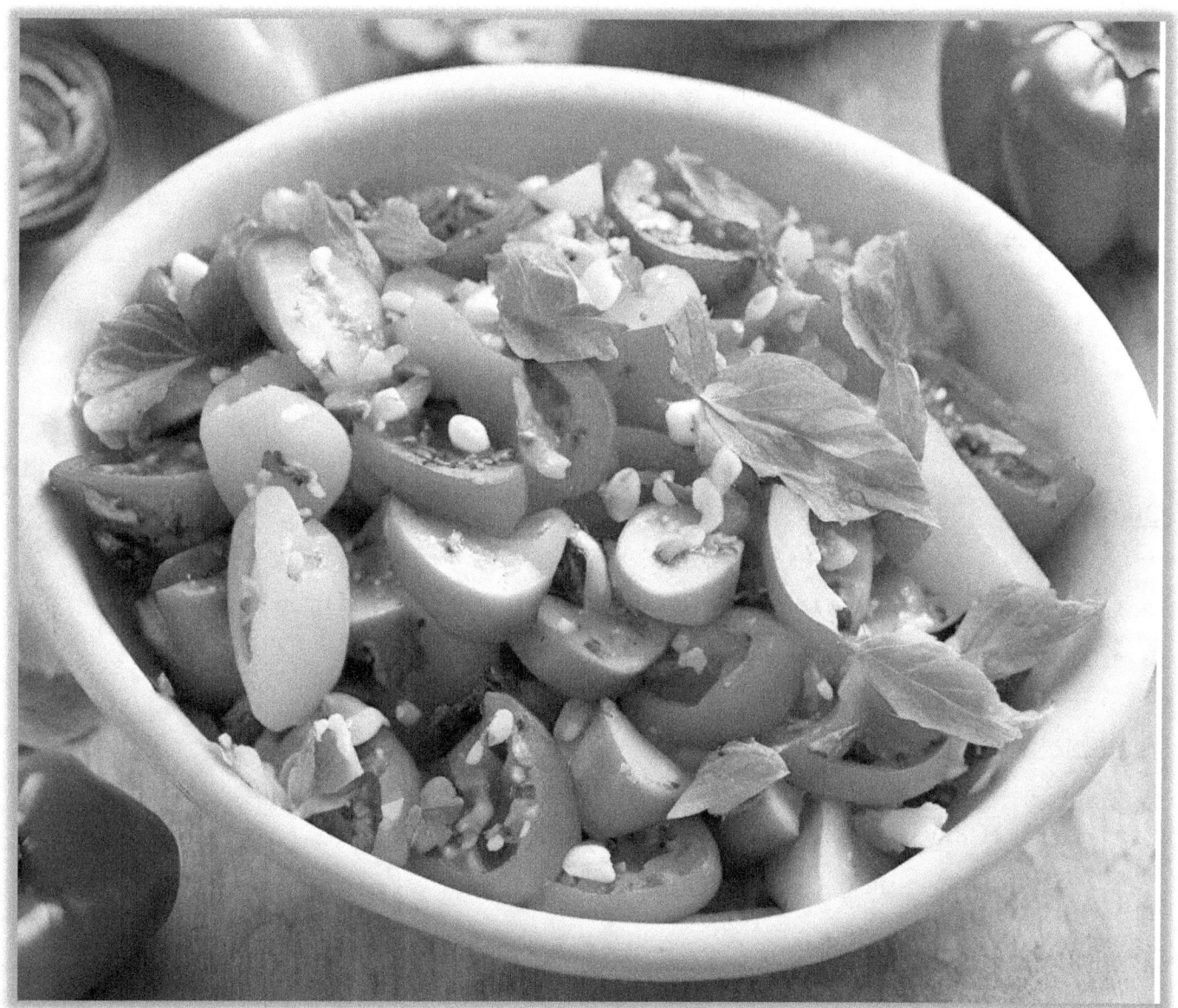

Main Dish Salad

Enjoy a nourishing and flavorful salad that keeps you satisfied as a complete dinner option! This recipe is packed with protein and lower-potassium vegetables, making it a perfect choice for those on a CKD diet.

PREP TIME: 15 MINUTES | COOK TIME: VARIES DEPENDING ON PROTEIN CHOICE (SEE BELOW) | YIELDS: 1 SERVING

INGREDIENTS:

Base:

- 2 cups mixed greens (such as romaine, spinach, or a combination)
- ½ cup chopped vegetables (such as cucumber, bell pepper, cherry tomatoes)

Protein Choice (pick one):

- 3 ounces grilled chicken breast, sliced
- 3 ounces baked salmon
- ½ cup cooked lentils or chickpeas (rinsed)

Other Optional Additions:

- ¼ cup crumbled low-fat feta cheese (potassium watch!) OR crumbled ricotta cheese
- ¼ cup chopped nuts or seeds (almonds, walnuts, sunflower seeds)

For the Dressing (choose one):

- Lemon Herb Vinaigrette (recipe below)
- Balsamic Vinaigrette (recipe below)

Lemon Herb Vinaigrette:

- 2 tablespoons olive oil
- 1 tablespoon lemon juice
- 1 teaspoon Dijon mustard (low-sodium option)
- ½ teaspoon dried oregano
- ¼ teaspoon dried thyme
- Pinch of garlic powder
- Salt-free herb seasoning (to taste)

Balsamic Vinaigrette:

- 2 tablespoons olive oil
- 1 tablespoon balsamic vinegar
- ½ teaspoon Dijon mustard (low-sodium option)
- Pinch of dried oregano
- Pinch of black pepper
- Salt-free herb seasoning (to taste)

COOKING INSTRUCTIONS:

1. Prepare your chosen protein according to package instructions or preferred method (grilling, baking, etc.). Cook lentils or chickpeas according to package directions if using.
2. In a large bowl, combine mixed greens, chopped vegetables, and your cooked protein.
3. Add any additional desired toppings like cheese or nuts/seeds.
4. In a separate small bowl, whisk together your chosen vinaigrette dressing (Lemon Herb or Balsamic).
5. Pour the dressing over the salad and toss to coat evenly.
6. Serve immediately and enjoy!

NUTRITIONAL INFORMATION: (APPROXIMATE VALUES PER SERVING, WILL VARY DEPENDING ON PROTEIN CHOICE)

Calories: 400-500 (depending on protein and additions)

Protein: 20-30 grams (depending on protein choice)

Potassium: 400mg (depending on vegetables and cheese)

Sodium: 50mg (depending on seasoning and cheese)

Phosphorus: 200mg (depending on protein choice)

TIPS FOR MODIFICATION:

- Protein Selection: Choose lean protein sources like grilled chicken or baked salmon for lower phosphorus content. If using lentils or chickpeas, consider portion size due to their phosphorus content.
- Dressing Choice: opt for the Lemon Herb Vinaigrette as it's generally lower in potassium than the Balsamic Vinaigrette. You can also use a store-bought low-sodium salad dressing.

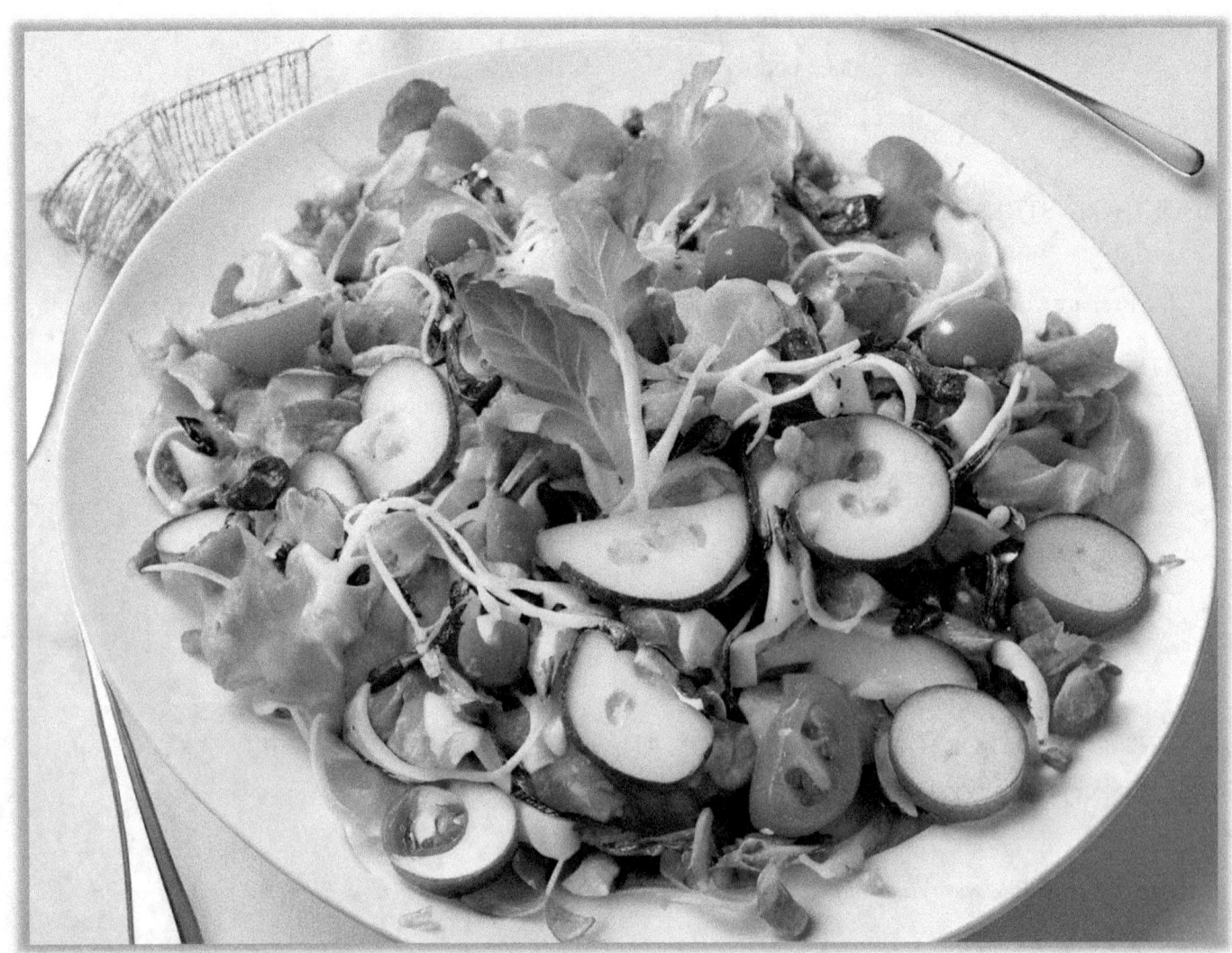

Ginger-Garlic Ramen Bowls

This recipe uses a lower-potassium vegetable broth and swaps traditional ramen noodles for a satisfying and kidney-friendly dinner.

PREP TIME: 10 MINUTES | COOK TIME: 15-20 MINUTES | YIELDS: 1 SERVING

INGREDIENTS:

- 1 cup low-sodium vegetable broth
- ½ cup chopped vegetables (broccoli florets, snap peas, carrots, etc.)
- 1 tablespoon olive oil
- ½ cup chopped onion
- 1 clove garlic, minced
- 1 teaspoon grated ginger
- ½ teaspoon low-sodium soy sauce (potassium watch!)
- ¼ teaspoon ground black pepper
- Optional protein (cooked and shredded chicken, tofu, etc.)
- Chopped green onions (for garnish)
- Salt-free herb seasoning (to taste)

COOKING INSTRUCTIONS:

1. In a medium saucepan, heat vegetable broth over medium heat. Add your chosen chopped vegetables and cook until tender-crisp (about 5 minutes).
2. While the vegetables cook, heat olive oil in a separate skillet over medium heat. Add chopped onion and cook until softened (2-3 minutes).
3. Stir in minced garlic and grated ginger, cook for an additional minute until fragrant.
4. Pour the cooked vegetables and broth from the saucepan into the skillet with the aromatics.
5. Add soy sauce, black pepper, and optional cooked protein (chicken, tofu, etc.) to the pot.
6. Bring to a simmer and cook for 2-3 minutes to heat through.
7. Taste and adjust seasonings with additional black pepper or a pinch of salt-free herb seasoning if desired.

8. Divide into a bowl and garnish with chopped green onions.

NUTRITIONAL INFORMATION: (APPROXIMATE VALUES PER SERVING)

Calories: 250 (depending on protein and vegetables)

Protein: 10 grams (depending on protein)

Potassium: 350mg (depending on vegetables)

Phosphorus: 80mg (depending on protein)

Sodium: 40mg (depending on seasoning)

TIPS FOR MODIFICATION:

- Potassium Control: Choose lower-potassium vegetables like green beans, zucchini, or cabbage. You can also rinse canned vegetables before using them.
- Protein Choice: opt for lean protein sources like shredded chicken or tofu for lower phosphorus content. Consider portion size and prioritize protein sources lower in phosphorus.

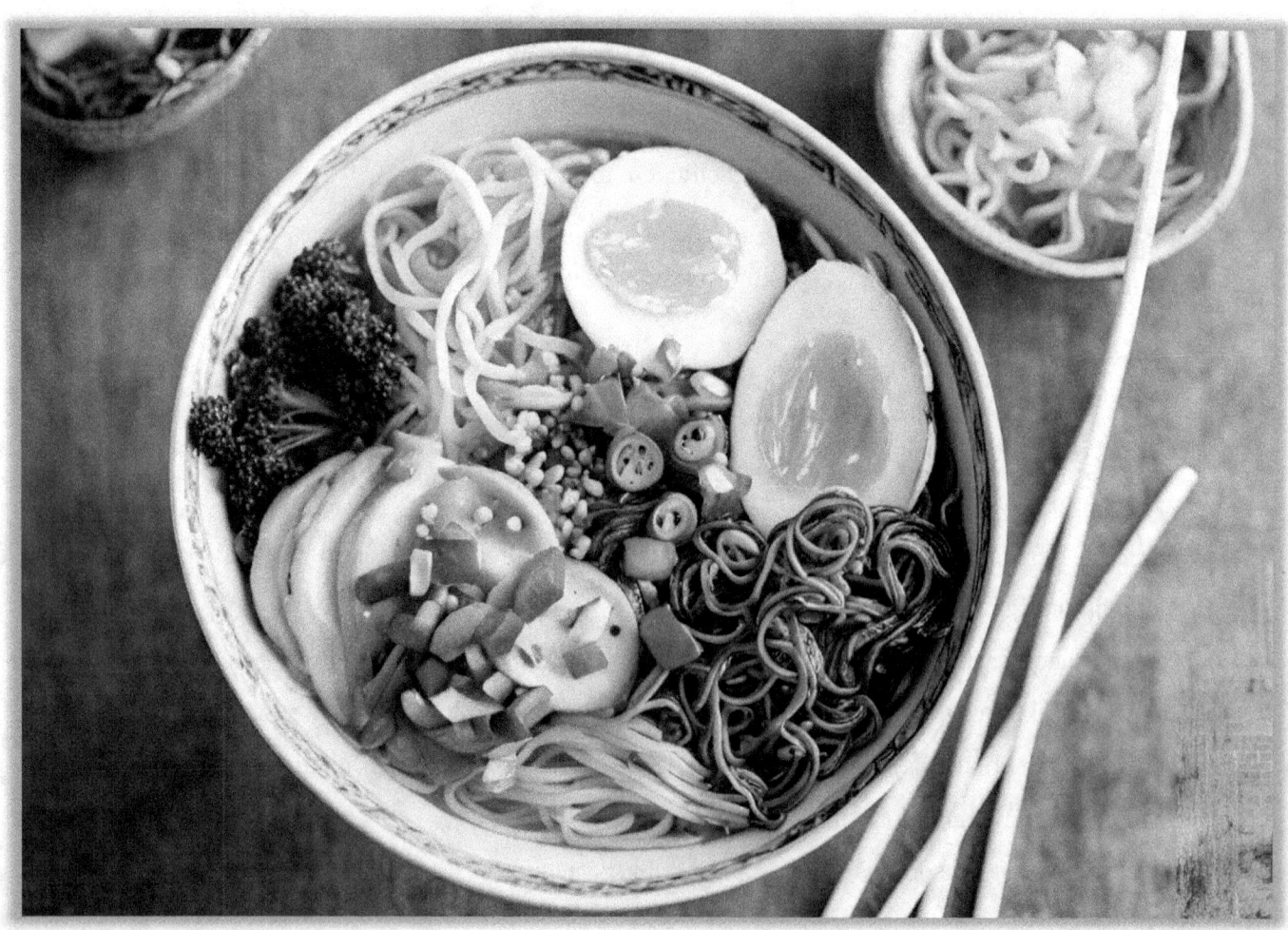

Tortilla-less Soup

This recipe is perfect for a CKD diet, featuring a flavorful broth packed with vegetables and shredded chicken, skipping the high-potassium tortillas for a kidney-friendly dinner.

PREP TIME: 10 MINUTES | COOK TIME: 15-20 MINUTES | YIELDS: 1 SERVING

INGREDIENTS:

- 1 cup low-sodium vegetable broth
- ½ cup chopped vegetables (corn, bell pepper, tomatoes, etc.) (potassium watch!)
- 1 tablespoon olive oil
- ½ cup chopped onion
- 1 clove garlic, minced
- 1 teaspoon chili powder
- ½ teaspoon ground cumin
- Pinch of smoked paprika (optional)
- 3 ounces cooked and shredded chicken breast
- Chopped fresh cilantro (for garnish)
- Salt-free herb seasoning (to taste)

COOKING INSTRUCTIONS:

1. In a medium saucepan, heat vegetable broth over medium heat. Add your chosen chopped vegetables and cook until tender-crisp (about 5 minutes). Potassium Control Tip: See tip #1 below for choosing lower-potassium vegetables.
2. While the vegetables cook, heat olive oil in a separate skillet over medium heat. Add chopped onion and cook until softened (2-3 minutes).
3. Stir in minced garlic and cook for an additional minute until fragrant.
4. Add chili powder, cumin, and smoked paprika (if using) to the skillet with the onions and cook for another minute, stirring constantly, to release the spices' flavors.
5. Pour the cooked vegetables and broth from the saucepan into the skillet with the spices.
6. Add cooked and shredded chicken breast to the pot.

7. Bring to a simmer and cook for 2-3 minutes to heat through.
8. Taste and adjust seasonings with additional spices or a pinch of salt-free herb seasoning if desired.
9. Serve hot in a bowl, garnished with chopped fresh cilantro.

NUTRITIONAL INFORMATION: (APPROXIMATE VALUES PER SERVING)

Calories: 300 (depending on vegetables)

Phosphorus: 200mg (depending on chicken)

Protein: 25 grams (from chicken)

Sodium: 50mg (depending on seasoning)

Potassium: 400mg (depending on vegetables)

TIPS FOR MODIFICATION:

- Potassium Control: Choose lower-potassium vegetables like green beans, zucchini, or mushrooms instead of corn, bell peppers, or tomatoes. Rinse canned vegetables before using them for further potassium reduction.
- Low-Carb Option: Skip the tortilla strips altogether for a more CKD-friendly meal. You can add a dollop of low-fat plain yogurt or sour cream for a touch of creaminess if desired.

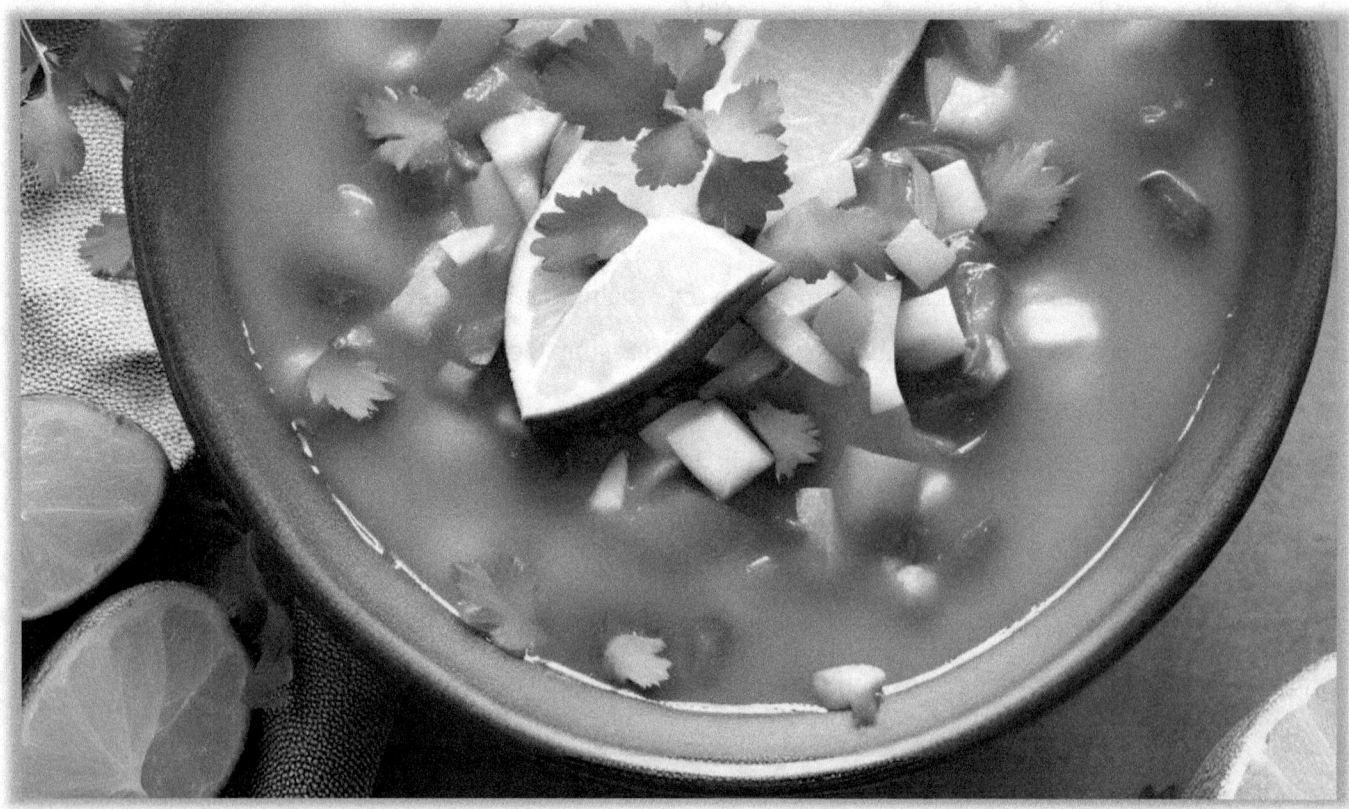

Smoky Caesar with Charred Romaine

Give classic Caesar salad a healthy twist! This recipe features romaine lettuce charred for a smoky flavor, all tossed in a lightened-up Caesar dressing for a satisfying and kidney-friendly dinner option.

PREP TIME: 10 MINUTES | COOK TIME: 5-7 MINUTES (DEPENDING ON CHARRING METHOD) | YIELDS: 1 SERVING

INGREDIENTS:

- 1 romaine lettuce heart, halved lengthwise
- 1 tablespoon olive oil
- Salt-free herb seasoning (to taste)
- For the CKD-Friendly Caesar Dressing:
- ¼ cup low-fat Greek yogurt
- 1 tablespoon low-fat mayonnaise
- 1 tablespoon lemon juice
- 1/2 anchovy fillet (or 1/2 teaspoon anchovy paste) (potassium watch!)
- 1 clove garlic, minced
- ½ teaspoon Dijon mustard (low-sodium option)
- Freshly ground black pepper (to taste)

COOKING INSTRUCTIONS:

1. Prepare the romaine: Drizzle romaine halves with olive oil and season with salt-free herb seasoning.
2. Char the romaine (choose one method):
3. Grill method: Preheat grill to medium-high heat. Grill romaine cut-side down for 2-3 minutes per side, or until slightly charred.
4. Skillet method: Heat a large skillet over medium-high heat. Add romaine halves, cut-side down, and cook for 2-3 minutes per side, or until slightly charred.

5. Make the dressing: In a small bowl, whisk together Greek yogurt, mayonnaise, lemon juice, anchovy fillet (or paste), garlic, Dijon mustard, and black pepper until smooth.
6. Assemble the salad: Place charred romaine halves on a plate. Drizzle with Caesar dressing and enjoy!

NUTRITIONAL INFORMATION: (APPROXIMATE VALUES PER SERVING)

Calories: 250

Phosphorus: 150mg

Protein: 10 grams (from yogurt)

Sodium: 100mg (depending on seasoning

Potassium: 250mg (depending on anchovy)

)

TIPS FOR MODIFICATION:

- Potassium Control: opt to omit the anchovy entirely or use a tiny amount. You can also use a splash of fish sauce instead, for a similar umami flavor without the potassium content.
- Lower Phosphorus: Choose a light mayonnaise option or use less mayonnaise overall. Consider adding a teaspoon of chopped fresh herbs like chives or dill for extra flavor.

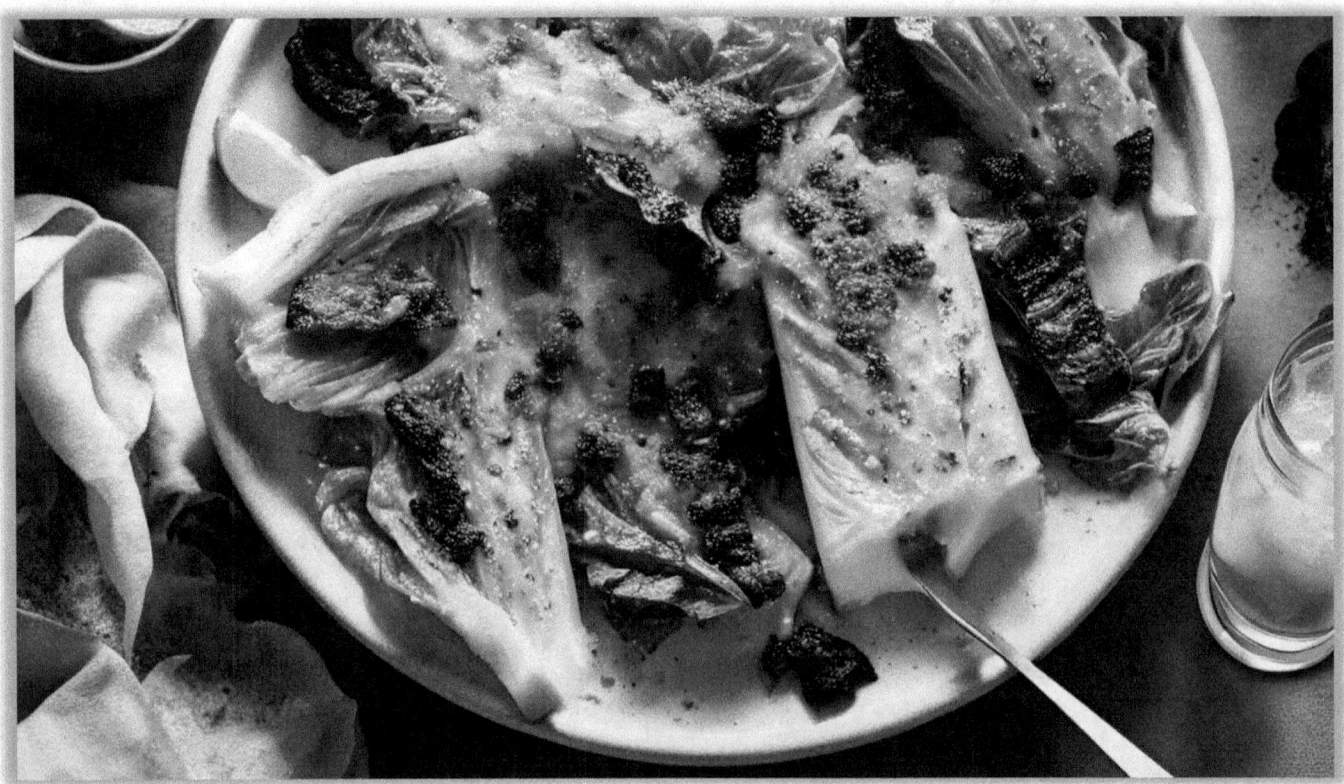

Jackfruit "Carnitas" Tacos

Enjoy a delicious and satisfying taco dinner that fits your CKD diet! This recipe uses jackfruit as a tasty substitute for traditional pork carnitas, simmered in a blend of spices for a flavor explosion. We've also made adjustments to lower the potassium and phosphorus content, making it a kidney-friendly meal.

PREP TIME: 15 MINUTES | COOK TIME: 20-25 MINUTES | YIELDS: 1 SERVING

INGREDIENTS:

- 1 cup canned young jackfruit in brine or water, rinsed and shredded
- 1 tablespoon olive oil
- 1/2 onion, diced
- 2 cloves garlic, minced
- 1 teaspoon chili powder
- 1/2 teaspoon cumin
- 1/4 teaspoon smoked paprika
- 1/4 cup low-sodium vegetable broth
- 1 tablespoon tomato paste
- 1/4 cup water
- 1 tablespoon lime juice (optional)
- Salt-free herb seasoning (to taste)
- 2 corn tortillas (or low-carb option like lettuce wraps) desired taco toppings (e.g. chopped cilantro, avocado slices)

COOKING INSTRUCTIONS:

1. Shred the jackfruit: Open the can of jackfruit, rinse well to remove brine flavor, and shred with your fingers or forks.
2. Heat oil in a large skillet over medium heat. Add the diced onion and cook until softened, about 3 minutes. Stir in the garlic and cook for an additional minute until fragrant.
3. Add the spices: Chili powder, cumin, and smoked paprika to the pan and cook for another minute, stirring constantly to release the flavors.

4. Pour in the vegetable broth, tomato paste, and water. Bring to a simmer and scrape up any browned bits from the bottom of the pan.
5. Add the jackfruit shreds and stir to coat. Season with a pinch of salt-free herb seasoning (to taste).
6. Simmer for 15-20 minutes, or until the jackfruit is tender and flavorful, stirring occasionally. Add a splash of water if the mixture seems too dry.
7. Taste and adjust seasonings with additional spices or lime juice (optional).
8. Warm your corn tortillas according to package instructions or your preferred method (microwave, stovetop, etc.). You can also use lettuce wraps for a low-carb option.
9. Fill your tortillas with jackfruit "carnitas" and your desired toppings like chopped cilantro and avocado slices. Enjoy!

NUTRITIONAL INFORMATION: (APPROXIMATE VALUES PER SERVING)

Calories: 400

Phosphorus: 150mg

Protein: 4 grams

Sodium: 50mg (depending on seasoning)

Potassium: 400mg (depending on vegetables)

TIPS FOR MODIFICATION:

- Lower Potassium: Choose low-potassium vegetables for toppings like shredded cabbage or chopped tomatoes. Rinse canned vegetables before using them for further potassium reduction.
- Portion Control: Be mindful of the amount of jackfruit you consume, as canned jackfruit can vary slightly in potassium content.

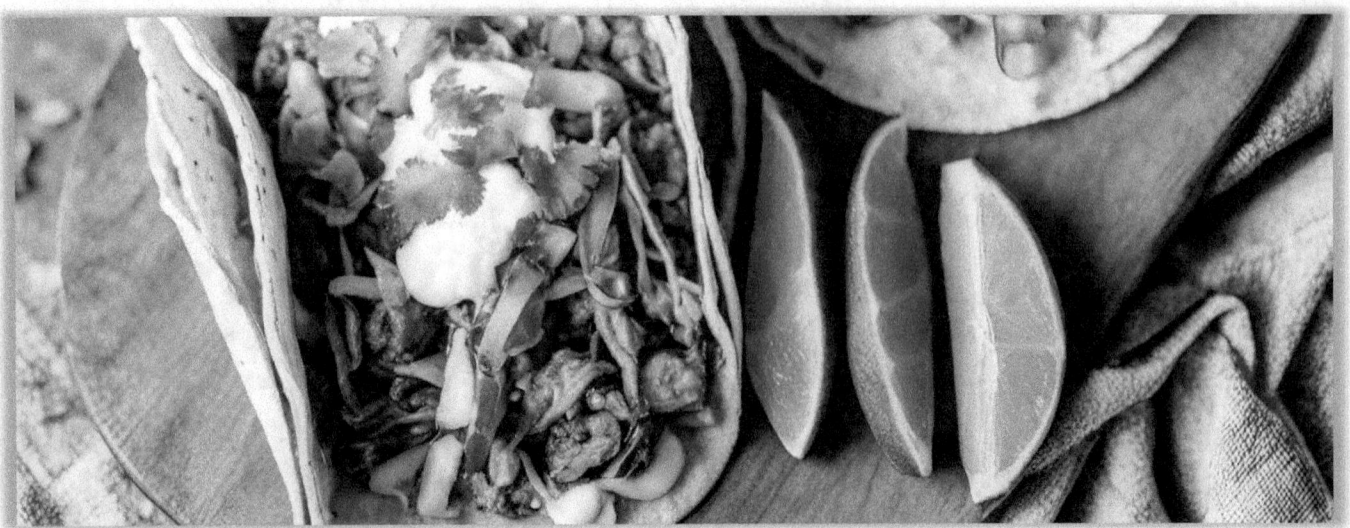

Watermelon Gazpacho

Beat the heat with a vibrant and flavorful watermelon gazpacho! Perfect for a light and satisfying CKD-friendly dinner, this chilled soup features refreshing watermelon with a touch of tomato and cucumber.

PREP TIME: 10 MINUTES | COOK TIME: NO COOK TIME (CHILLING RECOMMENDED) | YIELDS: 1 SERVING

INGREDIENTS:

- 2 cups cubed watermelon (fresh or canned in water, drained)
- ¼ cup chopped cucumber, peeled and seeded (optional)
- ¼ cup chopped tomato (optional)
- 1 tablespoon olive oil
- 1 tablespoon lemon juice
- ¼ teaspoon dried oregano
- Salt-free herb seasoning (to taste)
- Fresh mint or basil leaves (for garnish)

COOKING INSTRUCTIONS:

1. In a blender, combine cubed watermelon, chopped cucumber (if using), chopped tomato (if using), olive oil, lemon juice, and dried oregano.
2. Blend until smooth. Season with salt-free herb seasoning to taste.
3. Chill the gazpacho in the refrigerator for at least 30 minutes, or until cold.
4. Serve garnished with a fresh mint or basil leaf (optional).

NUTRITIONAL INFORMATION: (APPROXIMATE VALUES PER SERVING)

Calories: 150   *Potassium: 300mg (depending on vegetables)*

Protein: 1 gram   *Phosphorus: 40mg*

Sodium: 30mg (depending on seasoning)

TIPS FOR MODIFICATION:

- Potassium Control: opt for a smaller amount of cucumber and tomato, or skip them entirely, as they can be higher in potassium. You can focus primarily on the watermelon for a lower-potassium base.
- Low-Potassium Garnish: Skip the fresh mint or basil leaves as garnishes, or choose a very small amount. Chopped chives can be a good lower-potassium alternative.

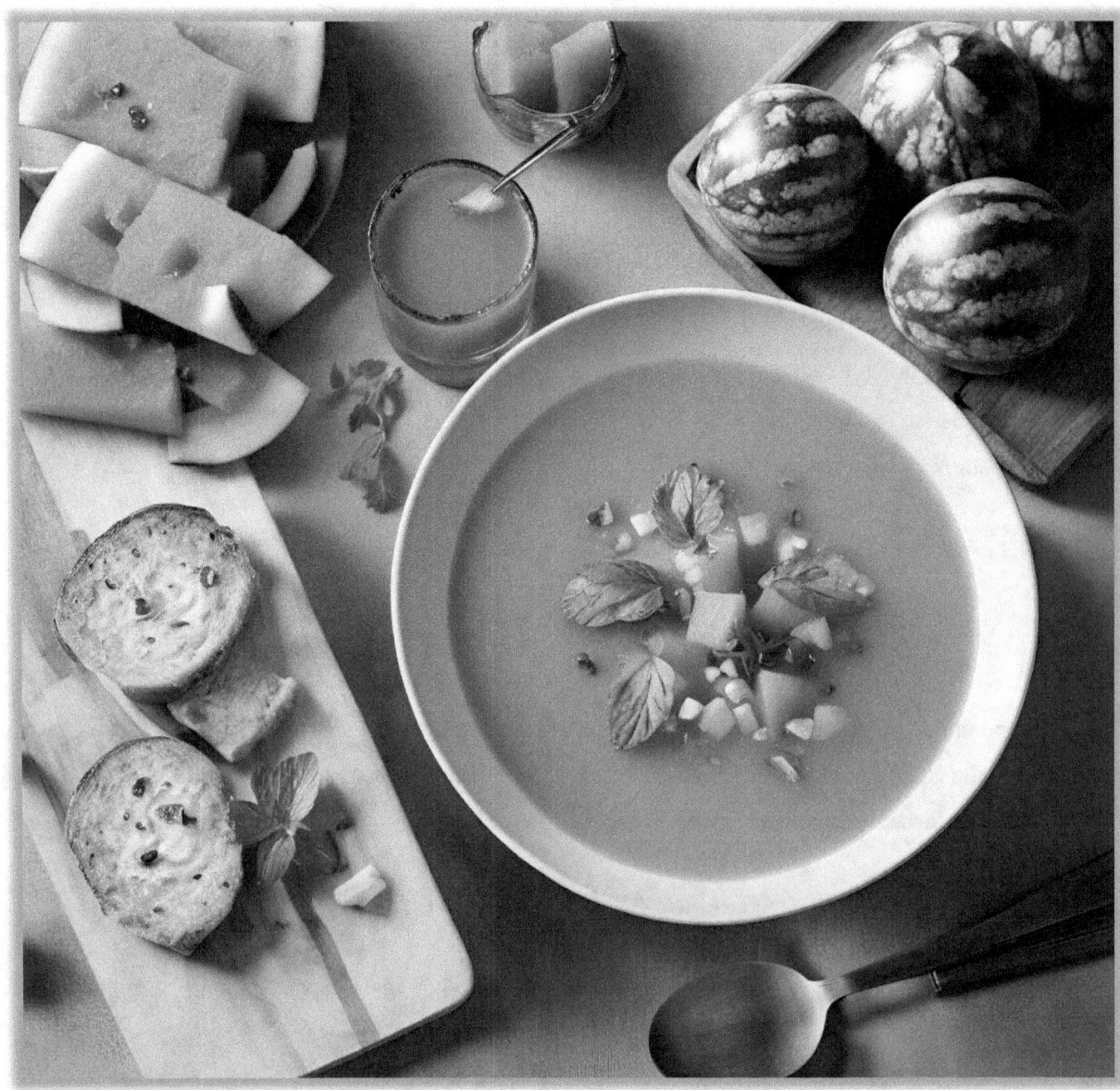

Mushroom Bourguignon

Enjoy the rich flavors of Bourguignon with a twist! This recipe uses mushrooms as the star ingredient, simmered in a flavorful red wine sauce. We've made adjustments to lower the phosphorus content, making it a perfect choice for a satisfying CKD dinner.

PREP TIME: 15 MINUTES | COOK TIME: 45-50 MINUTES | YIELDS: 1 SERVING

INGREDIENTS:

- 1 tablespoon olive oil
- 1 shallot, minced
- 1 clove garlic, minced
- 8 ounces assorted mushrooms (cremini, shiitake, portobello), sliced
- ½ cup low-sodium vegetable broth
- ¼ cup red wine (optional, you can substitute with more broth)
- 1 tablespoon tomato paste
- ½ teaspoon dried thyme
- Pinch of black pepper
- Salt-free herb seasoning (to taste)
- Chopped fresh parsley (for garnish, optional)

COOKING INSTRUCTIONS:

1. Heat olive oil in a large skillet over medium heat. Add shallot and cook until softened, about 3 minutes. Stir in garlic and cook for an additional minute until fragrant.
2. Add sliced mushrooms and cook for 5-7 minutes, or until softened and starting to release their juices.
3. Pour in vegetable broth, red wine (if using), tomato paste, thyme, and black pepper. Stir to scrape up any browned bits from the bottom of the pan.
4. Bring to a simmer and cook for 20-25 minutes, or until the sauce has thickened slightly.
5. Season with salt-free herb seasoning to taste.
6. Serve immediately garnished with chopped fresh parsley (optional).

NUTRITIONAL INFORMATION: (APPROXIMATE VALUES PER SERVING)

Calories: 250

Phosphorus: 200mg (depending on mushrooms)

Protein: 5 grams

Sodium: 50mg (depending on seasoning)

Potassium: 200mg (depending on vegetables)

TIPS FOR MODIFICATION:

- Phosphorus Management: Choose a mix of mushrooms lower in phosphorus, such as white button mushrooms or oyster mushrooms. Limit the amount of cremini or portobello mushrooms.
- Consider Bone Broth: For extra flavor, you can substitute a small amount of low-sodium chicken or beef bone broth for some of the vegetable broth. opt for a brand that specifies low phosphorus content.

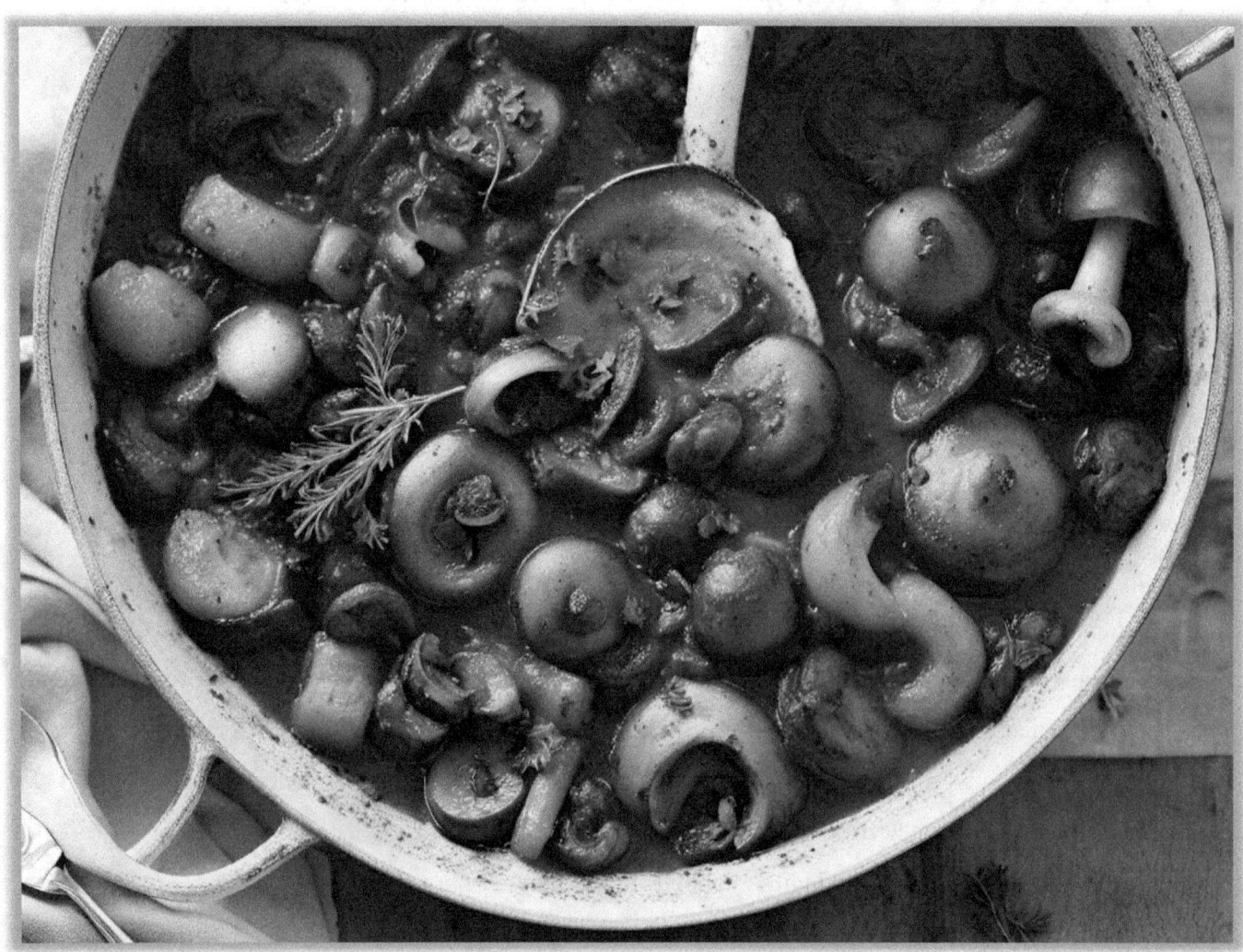

One-Pan Lemon Garlic Chicken with Veggies

This recipe for One-Pan Lemon Garlic Chicken with Veggies is packed with protein and features a simple lemon-garlic marinade that infuses the chicken with delicious taste. Plus, the vegetables roast alongside the chicken for a complete and hassle-free meal.

PREP TIME: 10 MINUTES | COOK TIME: 30 MINUTES | YIELDS: 1 SERVING

INGREDIENTS:

- 4 ounces boneless, skinless chicken breast
- 1 tablespoon olive oil
- ½ cup chopped vegetables (broccoli florets, asparagus spears, cherry tomatoes - choose lower potassium options like green beans or zucchini)
- ½ teaspoon dried oregano
- ¼ teaspoon garlic powder
- Pinch of black pepper
- ¼ cup low-sodium chicken broth
- 1 tablespoon lemon juice
- Salt-free herb seasoning (to taste)

COOKING INSTRUCTIONS:

1. Preheat oven to 400°F (200°C).
2. In a medium bowl, toss chicken breast with olive oil, oregano, garlic powder, and black pepper.
3. Arrange chicken in a single layer on a rimmed baking sheet. Scatter chosen chopped vegetables around the chicken.
4. Pour chicken broth and lemon juice into the bottom of the baking sheet.
5. Bake for 20-25 minutes, or until the chicken is cooked through and the vegetables are tender-crisp.
6. Season with salt-free herb seasoning to taste, if desired.

NUTRITIONAL INFORMATION: (APPROXIMATE VALUES PER SERVING)

Calories: 350

Phosphorus: 200mg

Protein: 30 grams

Sodium: 50mg (depending on seasoning)

Potassium: 300mg (depending on vegetables)

TIPS FOR MODIFICATION:

- For extra flavor, marinate the chicken in the olive oil, herbs, and spices for 15-30 minutes before baking.
- You can adjust the vegetables based on your preferences and what's lower in potassium.
- Consider adding a sprinkle of low-sodium parmesan cheese on top of the chicken for the last few minutes of baking for a touch of cheesy flavor.

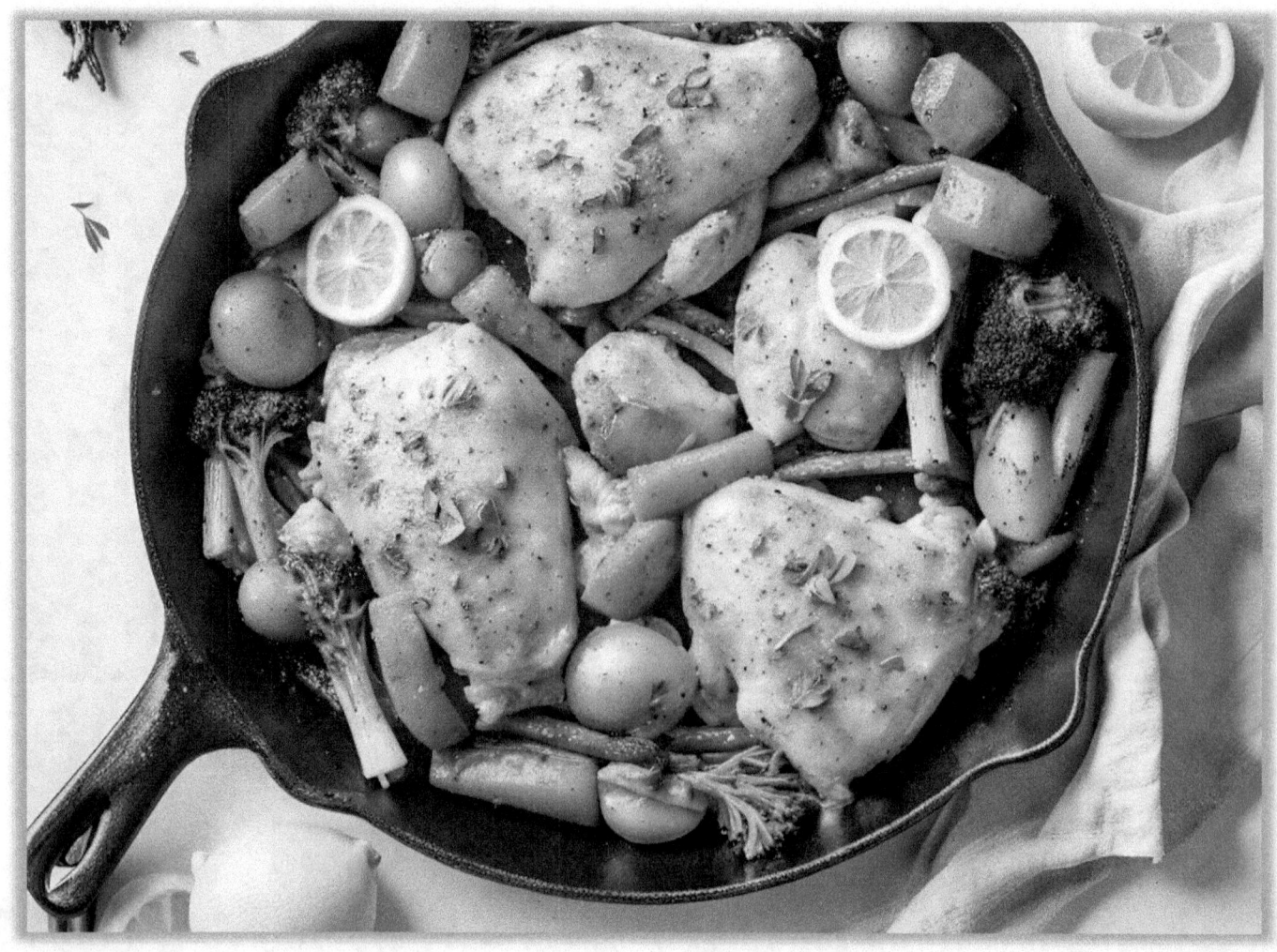

SANCK OPTIONS

You have been doing an amazing job navigating the world of kidney-friendly meals, and now it's time for the fun part: snacks! Who says you can't have a little crunch, a little sweetness, and a whole lot of flavors while keeping your kidneys happy? This section is packed with snack recipes that are low in protein, potassium, sodium, and phosphorus, but high on deliciousness.

Tips for Making the Most of These Recipes

1. Preparation is Key: Think of yourself as a snacking ninja—always ready with a healthy treat! A little prep work goes a long way. Get those snacks ready in advance so you can avoid the temptation of less nutritious options.
2. Portion Control: Remember, even the yummiest snacks need to be enjoyed in moderation. Stick to the recommended serving sizes to keep things balanced and your kidneys smiling.
3. Ingredient Substitutions: Don't sweat it if you don't have every ingredient on hand. Feel free to swap out for other kidney-friendly options that you like. Creativity in the kitchen is highly encouraged!
4. Balance and Variety: Variety is the spice of life, and your taste buds will thank you for mixing things up. Try different snacks throughout the week to keep things exciting and nutritionally balanced.

What to Expect

- Creamy and Crunchy Combos: Get ready for some seriously satisfying textures with snacks like Curd & Crunch Cottage Cheese and Crunchy Carrot and Creamy Hummus Delight. These combos will have you crunching and munching happily.
- Light and Sweet Treats: Craving something sweet? Indulge in Light and Sweet Yogurt Parfait and Creamy Cottage Cheese & Berry Delight. These treats are so good, you'll feel like you're having dessert.
- Savory and Satisfying: For those moments when you need something savory, reach for Veggie Straw, Hard-Boiled Delight, and Air-Popped Popcorn Perfection. Perfect for any time of the day when the munchies strike.

- Fresh and Fruity: Enjoy the natural sweetness of fruits with Rice Cake Remix, Almonds and Apple, and Berry Blast Smoothie. These snacks are refreshing and packed with vitamins—your body will thank you.
- Fun and Flavorful: Spice things up with Mini Veggie Skewers and Edamame Energy, These snacks are not just tasty, they're fun to make and eat!

Go ahead, dive into these recipes, and make snacking a delightful, nutritious part of your day. Keep up the fantastic work—you've got this!

Curd and Crunch Cottage Cheese

Sometimes you just need a quick and protein-packed snack! This recipe features creamy cottage cheese with refreshing cucumber for a satisfying and kidney-friendly option.

PREP TIME: 5 MINUTES | COOK TIME: NO COOK TIME | YIELDS: 1 SERVING

INGREDIENTS:

- ¼ cup cottage cheese
- ½ cup sliced cucumber
- ¼ teaspoon dried dill (optional)

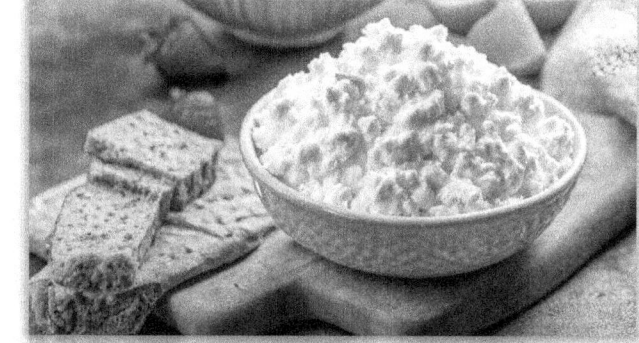

COOKING INSTRUCTIONS:

1. In a small bowl, combine ¼ cup cottage cheese and ½ cup sliced cucumber.
2. Sprinkle with ¼ teaspoon dried dill (optional) for additional flavor.
3. Enjoy!

NUTRITIONAL INFORMATION: (APPROXIMATE VALUES PER SERVING)

Calories: 100

Phosphorus: 150mg

Protein: 12 grams

Sodium: 80mg (depending on cheese)

Potassium: 200mg (depending on vegetables)

TIPS FOR MODIFICATION:

- Potassium Control: Choose low-sodium cottage cheese to further reduce potassium content.
- Flavor Boost: Experiment with different herbs or spices like chives or garlic powder for additional flavor variations.

Carrot and Creamy Hummus

Enjoy a satisfying combination of crunchy carrots and creamy hummus for a quick and protein-packed snack! This recipe is perfect for satisfying your sweet and savory cravings while following your CKD diet.

PREP TIME: 2 MINUTES | COOK TIME: NO COOK TIME | YIELDS: 1 SERVING

INGREDIENTS:

- 2 baby carrots
- 2 tablespoons hummus

COOKING INSTRUCTIONS:

1. Wash and scrub the baby carrots.
2. Slice the baby carrots into sticks or your desired shape.

NUTRITIONAL INFORMATION: (APPROXIMATE VALUES PER SERVING)

Calories: 150

Phosphorus: 80mg

Protein: 4 grams

Sodium: 60mg (depending on hummus)

Potassium: 200mg (depending on vegetables)

TIPS FOR MODIFICATION:

- Potassium Control: Choose baby carrots over larger carrots, as they tend to be lower in potassium.
- Lower Sodium Hummus: opt for low-sodium hummus to further reduce sodium content.

Sweet Yogurt Parfait

Craving a sweet treat that fits your CKD diet? This yogurt parfait is a delicious and satisfying option with a controlled portion size. Packed with protein and a touch of fruit, it's the perfect way to curb your sweet tooth without compromising your kidney health.

PREP TIME: 5 MINUTES | COOK TIME: NO COOK TIME | YIELDS: 1 SERVING

INGREDIENTS:

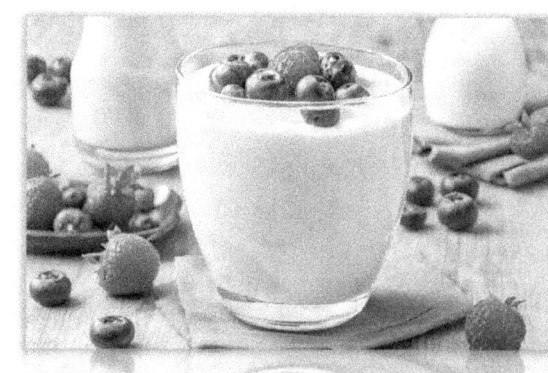

- ¼ cup plain Greek yogurt (low-fat option)
- 2 tablespoons sliced strawberries or blueberries
- Sprinkle of granola (limited portion)

COOKING INSTRUCTIONS:

1. In a small bowl or parfait glass, layer ¼ cup of plain Greek yogurt.
2. Top the yogurt with 2 tablespoons of your chosen sliced fruit (strawberries or blueberries).
3. Finish with a sprinkle of granola for added texture and flavor.

NUTRITIONAL INFORMATION: (APPROXIMATE VALUES PER SERVING)

Calories: 150

Phosphorus: 100mg

Protein: 10 grams (from yogurt)

Sodium: 40mg (depending on yogurt)

Potassium: 50mg (depending on fruit)

<u>TIPS FOR MODIFICATION:</u>

- Portion Control: Use a limited amount of granola to keep phosphorus content in check. Consider a sprinkle for added flavor and texture.
- Berry Choice: opt for berries lower in potassium like blueberries or raspberries instead of bananas or mangoes.

Veggie Straw

Sometimes you just need a quick and satisfying crunch! Veggie straws offer a convenient snack option that can fit into your CKD diet.

PREP TIME: 1 MINUTE | COOK TIME: NO COOK TIME | YIELDS: 1 SERVING

INGREDIENTS:

- 1 cup veggie straws (made from vegetables like carrots or beets)

COOKING INSTRUCTIONS:

1. Open a package of veggie straws (made from your preferred vegetables).
2. Enjoy 1 cup of veggie straws for a satisfying and crunchy snack.

NUTRITIONAL INFORMATION: (APPROXIMATE VALUES PER SERVING)

Calories: 100

Phosphorus: 40mg

Protein: 1 gram

Sodium: 30mg (depending on seasoning)

Potassium: 200mg (depending on vegetables)

TIPS FOR MODIFICATION:

- Variety is Key: Choose veggie straws made from a variety of vegetables for a wider range of nutrients and potentially lower potassium content.
- Portion Control: While generally lower in potassium than potato chips, monitor your intake to manage potassium content.

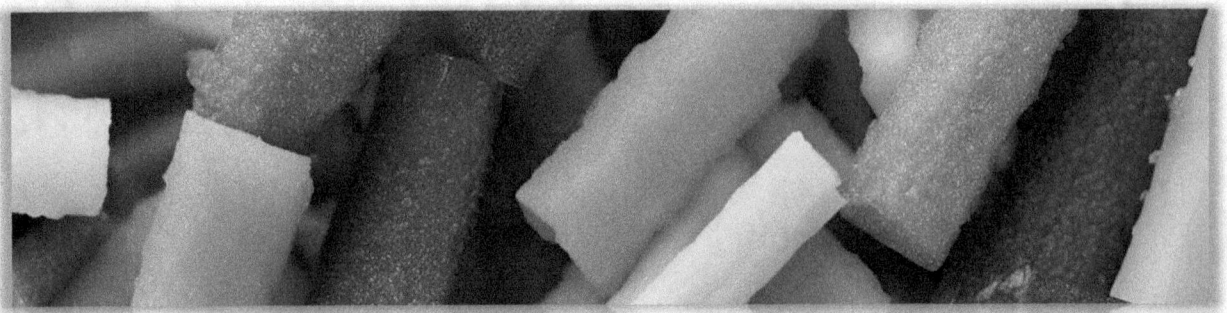

Creamy Cottage Cheese & Berry

Enjoy a delightful combination of creamy cottage cheese and fresh berries for a quick and satisfying snack! This recipe is perfect for a sweet treat that fits your CKD diet.

PREP TIME: 5 MINUTES | COOK TIME: NO COOK TIME | YIELDS: 1 SERVING

INGREDIENTS:

- ¼ cup cottage cheese
- ¼ cup chopped strawberries or raspberries

COOKING INSTRUCTIONS:

1. In a small bowl, combine ¼ cup cottage cheese and your chosen chopped berries (strawberries or raspberries).
2. Stir gently to combine.

NUTRITIONAL INFORMATION: (APPROXIMATE VALUES PER SERVING)

Calories: 100

Phosphorus: 130mg

Protein: 12 grams (from cottage cheese)

Sodium: 80mg (depending on cheese)

Potassium: 150mg (depending on fruit)

TIPS FOR MODIFICATION:

- Berry Choice: opt for berries lower in potassium like blueberries or raspberries instead of bananas or mangoes.
- Portion Control: Enjoy the full amount of cottage cheese for protein, but consider using slightly less fruit (2-3 tablespoons) to manage potassium intake.

Rice Cake

Turn a simple rice cake into a flavorful and satisfying snack option! This recipe features a creamy avocado topping with fresh chives for a delicious and kidney-friendly twist.

PREP TIME: 5 MINUTES | COOK TIME: NO COOK TIME | YIELDS: 1 SERVING

INGREDIENTS:

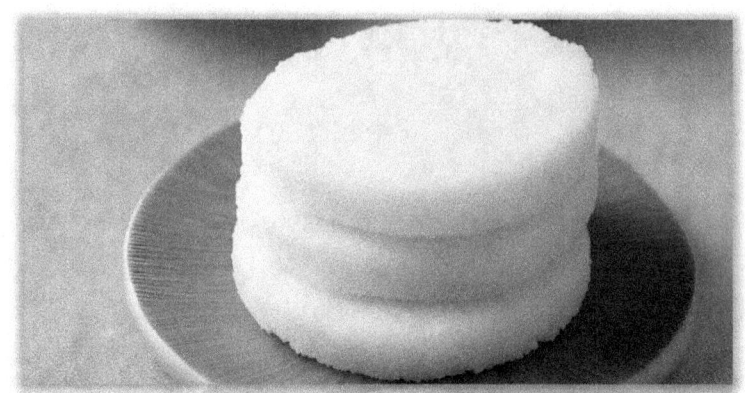

- 1 small brown rice cake
- 1 tablespoon mashed avocado
- Sprinkle of chopped fresh chives

COOKING INSTRUCTIONS:

1. Mash 1 tablespoon of avocado with a fork until creamy.
2. Spread the mashed avocado evenly over the small brown rice cake.
3. Sprinkle with chopped fresh chives for added flavor.

NUTRITIONAL INFORMATION: (APPROXIMATE VALUES PER SERVING)

Calories: 150

Phosphorus: 80mg

Protein: 2 grams

Sodium: 30mg (depending on cheese)

Potassium: 100mg (depending on avocado)

TIPS FOR MODIFICATION:

- Potassium Control: Choose a smaller brown rice cake to manage overall portion size and potassium intake.
- Avocado Choice: opt for a ripe avocado as it will be easier to mash and potentially lower in potassium content.

Air-Popped Popcorn

Air-popped popcorn is a satisfying and kidney-friendly option that's low in fat and phosphorus.

PREP TIME: 5 MINUTES | COOK TIME: 5-7 MINUTES | YIELDS: 1 SERVING

INGREDIENTS:

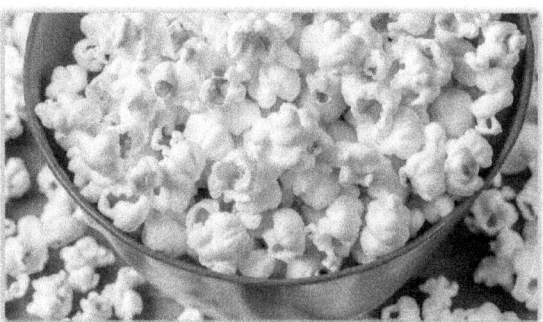

- 3 cups air-popped popcorn kernels
- Sprinkle of olive oil (optional)
- Dried herbs (like rosemary or thyme, optional)

COOKING INSTRUCTIONS:

1. Heat a large pot with a lid over medium heat. If using olive oil, add a few drops to coat the bottom of the pot.
2. Add the popcorn kernels to the pot in a single layer (avoid overcrowding).
3. Cover the pot with the lid and listen for the kernels popping. Shake the pot occasionally to prevent burning.
4. Once the popping slows down significantly (with a few seconds between pops), remove the pot from the heat.
5. Transfer the popcorn to a bowl and season with a sprinkle of olive oil (optional) and your chosen dried herbs (optional) for added flavor.

NUTRITIONAL INFORMATION: (APPROXIMATE VALUES PER SERVING)

Calories: 150

Phosphorus: 40mg

Protein: 3 grams

Sodium: 30mg (depending on seasoning)

Potassium: 100mg

TIPS FOR MODIFICATION:

- Skip the Oil: Air-popped popcorn is naturally low in fat. You can enjoy it plain or with a minimal amount of olive oil for additional flavor.
- Spice it Up: Experiment with different dried herbs or low-sodium seasonings to add variety to your popcorn snack.

Mini Veggie Skewers

This recipe is packed with nutrients and perfect for portion control, making it a great choice for a satisfying CKD-friendly snack.

PREP TIME: 5 MINUTES | COOK TIME: NO COOK TIME (OPTIONAL) | YIELDS: 1 SERVING

INGREDIENTS:

- Cherry tomatoes
- Bell pepper (choose green or yellow) cubes
- Sugar snap peas
- Low-sodium cheese cubes (optional)
- Skewers

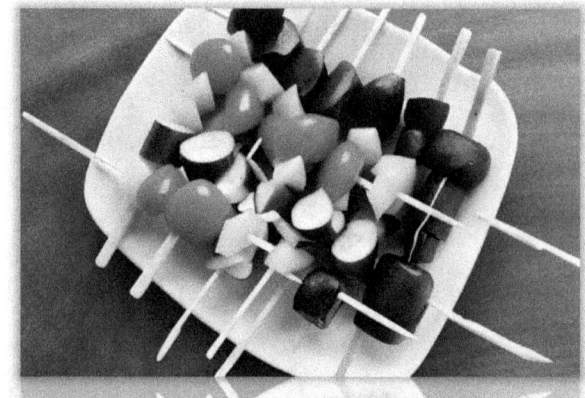

COOKING INSTRUCTIONS:

1. Wash and prepare your chosen vegetables: cherry tomatoes, green or yellow bell pepper cubes, and sugar snap peas.
2. Thread the vegetables onto skewers in a desired pattern. You can alternate colors for a more vibrant look.
3. If using low-sodium cheese cubes, add them to the skewers in between the vegetables (optional).

NUTRITIONAL INFORMATION: (APPROXIMATE VALUES PER SERVING)

Calories: 50 (without cheese) 80 (with cheese)

Phosphorus: 40mg

Protein: 2 grams (with cheese)

Sodium: 30mg (depending on cheese)

Potassium: 200mg (depending on vegetables)

TIPS FOR MODIFICATION:

- Vegetable Choice: opt for green or yellow bell peppers, as they tend to be lower in potassium than other colors.
- Cheese or No Cheese: Enjoy the skewers plain for a lower phosphorus content. If using cheese, choose a low-sodium option and limit the quantity.

Edamame Energy

Need a quick and protein-packed energy boost? Look no further than edamame! This recipe features simply steamed soybeans for a satisfying and kidney-friendly snack.

PREP TIME: 2 MINUTES | COOK TIME: 4-5 MINUTES | YIELDS: 1 SERVING

INGREDIENTS:

- ½ cup shelled edamame

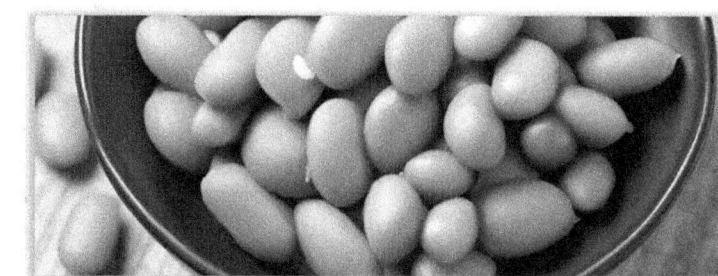

COOKING INSTRUCTIONS:

1. In a small saucepan, add ½ cup of shelled edamame and enough water to cover them.
2. Bring the water to a boil over high heat.
3. Once boiling, reduce heat and simmer for 4-5 minutes, or until the edamame are tender-crisp.
4. Drain the edamame in a colander and rinse under cold running water to stop the cooking process.
5. Season with a sprinkle of salt-free herb seasoning (optional) for added flavor.

NUTRITIONAL INFORMATION: (APPROXIMATE VALUES PER SERVING)

Calories: 120

Phosphorus: 180mg

Protein: 12 grams

Sodium: 15mg

Potassium: 150mg

TIPS FOR MODIFICATION:

- Portion Control: Edamame is a good source of plant-based protein but higher in phosphorus than some options. Enjoy a moderate serving size to manage phosphorus intake.
- Skip the Salt: Edamame is naturally flavorful. Use salt-free herb seasoning or enjoy it plain to keep sodium intake in check.

Almonds and Apple

Enjoy a satisfying mix of healthy fats and protein with this Nutty Delight recipe! Almonds offer a satisfying crunch, while apples add a touch of sweetness for a balanced and kidney-friendly snack.

PREP TIME: 2 MINUTES | COOK TIME: NO COOK TIME | YIELDS: 1 SERVING

INGREDIENTS:

- ¼ cup unsalted almonds
- 1 apple (sliced)

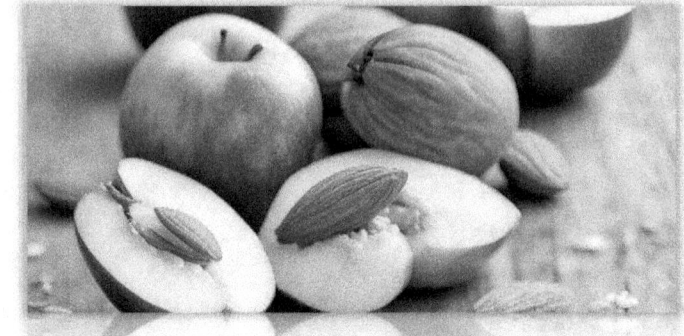

COOKING INSTRUCTIONS:

1. In a small bowl, combine ¼ cup of unsalted almonds and sliced apple.

NUTRITIONAL INFORMATION: (APPROXIMATE VALUES PER SERVING)

Calories: 200

Phosphorus: 150mg

Protein: 6 grams (from almonds)

Sodium: 30mg (depending on ingredients

Potassium: 200mg (depending on fruit)

)

TIPS FOR MODIFICATION:

- Nut Choice: While almonds are a good option, consider lower-potassium nuts like macadamia nuts or pecans for an alternative.
- Portion Control: Enjoy a moderate serving size to manage potassium and phosphorus content.

Berry Blast Smoothie

Craving a refreshing and satisfying snack? This Berry Blast Smoothie is packed with antioxidants and made with lower-potassium ingredients for a delicious CKD-friendly option.

PREP TIME: 5 MINUTES | COOK TIME: NO COOK TIME | YIELDS: 1 SERVING

INGREDIENTS:

- ½ cup frozen blueberries or raspberries
- ½ cup unsweetened almond milk (or other low-potassium milk option)
- ¼ cup plain Greek yogurt (low-fat option)
- Optional: Sugar substitute (to taste)
- Optional: Ice cubes

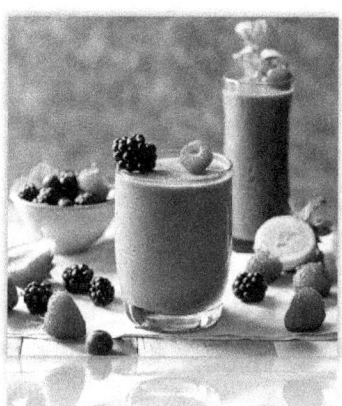

COOKING INSTRUCTIONS:

1. In a blender, combine ½ cup of frozen blueberries or raspberries, ½ cup of unsweetened almond milk (or other low-potassium milk option), and ¼ cup of plain Greek yogurt (low-fat option).
2. Blend until smooth and creamy.
3. Taste the smoothie and add sugar substitute (if using) to achieve your desired level of sweetness.
4. Add ice cubes (optional) for an extra refreshing drink.

NUTRITIONAL INFORMATION: (APPROXIMATE VALUES PER SERVING)

Calories: 150

Phosphorus: 100mg

Protein: 8 grams (from yogurt)

Sodium: 40mg (depending on yogurt)

Potassium: 150mg (depending on fruit)

TIPS FOR MODIFICATION:

- Berry Choice: Blueberries and raspberries are generally lower in potassium than some other berries.
- Milk Choice: Unsweetened almond milk is a lower-potassium option compared to cow's milk. You can explore other low-potassium milk options like oat milk or coconut milk.

Feta and Dill Cucumber Refreshers

Enjoy a refreshing and satisfying crunch with this Savory Cucumber Delight recipe! This simple snack is packed with flavor and moisture, making it a perfect choice for a hot day or whenever you need a light and kidney-friendly bite.

PREP TIME: 2 MINUTES | COOK TIME: NO COOK TIME | YIELDS: 1 SERVING

INGREDIENTS:

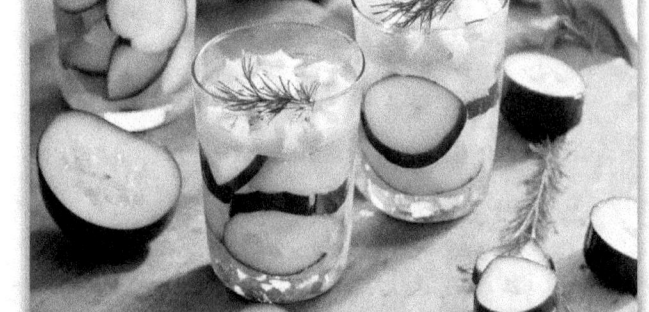

- 1 large cucumber
- 1 tablespoon crumbled low-fat feta cheese
- Pinch of dried dill weed
- Black pepper (to taste)

COOKING INSTRUCTIONS:

1. Wash and dry the cucumber. Slice the cucumber into rounds or sticks, whichever you prefer.
2. In a small bowl, combine the cucumber slices with crumbled low-fat feta cheese.
3. Sprinkle with dried dill weed and black pepper to taste.

NUTRITIONAL INFORMATION: (APPROXIMATE VALUES PER SERVING)

Calories: 30

Phosphorus: 40mg

Protein: 2 grams (from feta cheese)

Sodium: 150mg (depending on feta cheese)

Potassium: 200mg

TIPS FOR MODIFICATION:

- Portion Control: Monitor your feta cheese intake to manage sodium content.
- Herb Options: Explore other low-potassium herbs like parsley or oregano for a flavor variation.

MAIN COURSES

Welcome to the Main Courses! Here, you'll find a variety of mouth-watering recipes that cater to all your dining preferences, whether you're a meat lover, seafood enthusiast, or soup and salad aficionado. Each recipe is meticulously crafted to be low in protein, potassium, sodium, and phosphorus.

Tips for Making the Most of These Recipes

1. **Preparation is Key:** The secret to a stress-free cooking experience is preparation. Gather all your ingredients and measure them out before you start cooking. This will make the cooking process smoother and more enjoyable.
2. **Portion Control:** Sticking to the recommended serving sizes ensures you get the right balance of nutrients without overloading on protein, potassium, sodium, or phosphorus. This is crucial for maintaining your kidney health.
3. **Substitutions and Adjustments:** Feel free to make substitutions that align with your taste and dietary needs. For example, swap out high-potassium vegetables for lower-potassium alternatives, or use herbs and spices to enhance flavor without adding extra sodium.
4. **Balance and Variety:** Mix and match recipes from different sections to create balanced meals. Pairing a hearty meat dish with a light salad or soup can provide a satisfying and nutritious dining experience.

What to Expect

In this section, you'll discover a wide array of delicious and kidney-friendly main course recipes. Expect to find:

1. **Flavorful Meat and Fish Dishes:** Enjoy a variety of hearty, savory options like Garlic Herb Roasted Chicken, Skillet Steak with Chimichurri, and Blackened Tilapia with Cajun Seasoning, all designed to be low in protein, potassium, sodium, and phosphorus.
2. **Comforting Soups and Refreshing Salads:** Warm up with nutritious soups like Chicken and Vegetable Soup and Taco Soup with Ground Beef, or cool down with crisp salads such as Grilled Chicken Caesar Salad and Salmon Salad with Berries and Walnuts.

MEAT AND FISH

Garlic Herb Roasted Chicken

Packed with protein and easy to prepare, this dish is perfect for a satisfying CKD-friendly meal.

PREP TIME: 10 MINUTES | COOK TIME: 1 HOUR | YIELDS: 4 SERVINGS

INGREDIENTS:

- 1 whole roasting chicken (about 4-5 lbs.)
- 2 tablespoons olive oil
- 2 tablespoons chopped fresh rosemary (or 1 teaspoon dried)
- 2 tablespoons chopped fresh thyme (or 1 teaspoon dried)
- 4 cloves garlic, minced
- 1 lemon, halved
- ½ teaspoon black pepper
- Salt (optional, to taste)

COOKING INSTRUCTIONS:

1. Preheat oven to 425°F (220°C).
2. In a small bowl, combine olive oil, rosemary, thyme, garlic, and black pepper.
3. Pat the chicken dry with paper towels. Rub the herb mixture all over the chicken, including under the skin. Season the cavity with a pinch of pepper (optional, and salt to taste if desired).
4. Place the chicken in a roasting pan and tuck the lemon halves into the cavity.
5. Roast the chicken for 1 hour, or until the internal temperature reaches 165°F (74°C) in the thickest part of the thigh. Baste the chicken with pan drippings occasionally for extra flavor.
6. Let the chicken rest for 10 minutes before carving and serving.

NUTRITIONAL INFORMATION: (APPROXIMATE VALUES PER SERVING)

Calories: 400

Potassium: 200mg (depending on portion size)

Protein: 50 grams

Phosphorus: 250mg

Sodium: 60mg (depending on added salt)

TIPS FOR MODIFICATION:

- Skin Removal: Consider removing the skin before cooking to reduce fat content.
- Potassium Management: Monitor portion size to manage overall potassium intake.

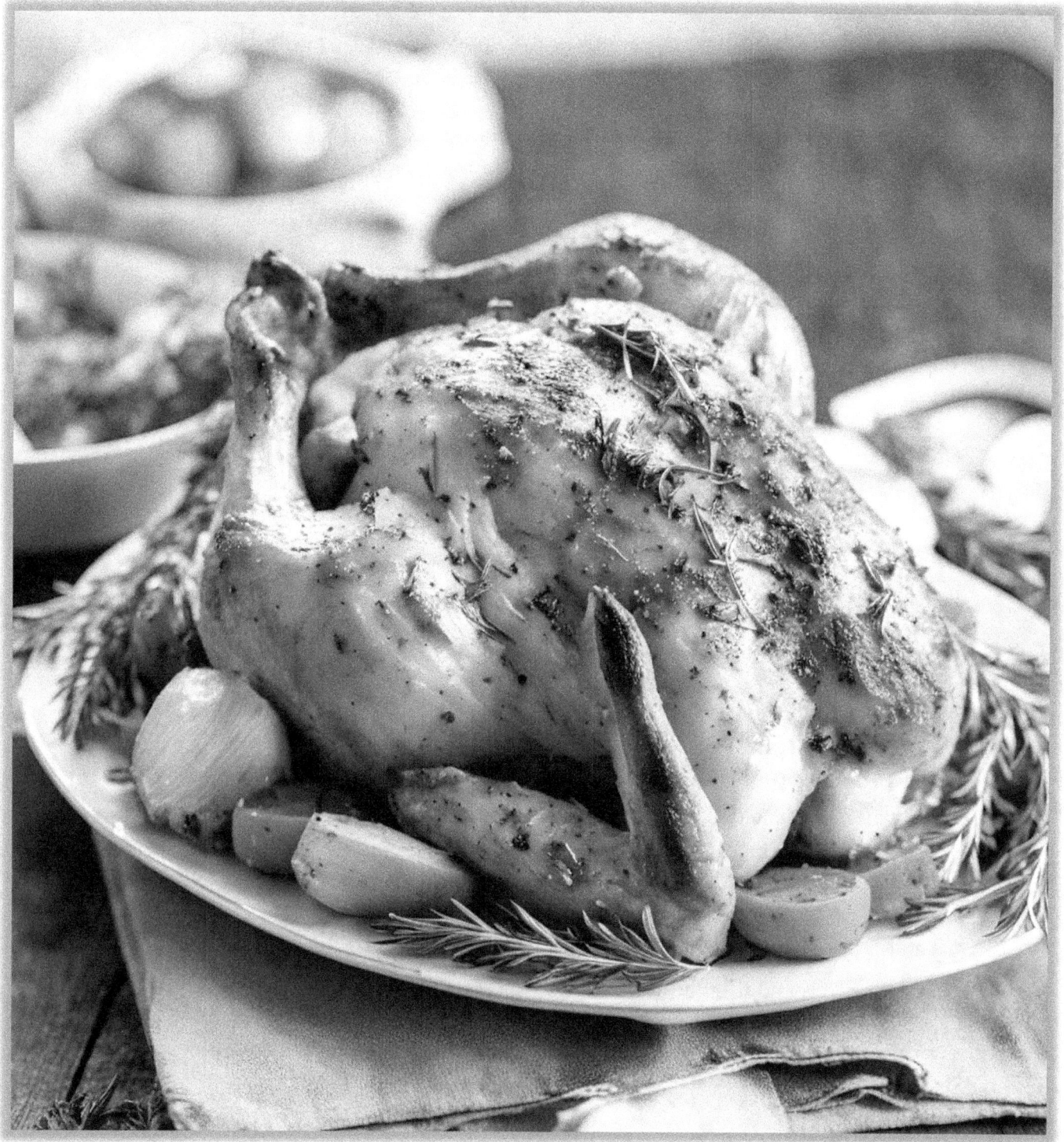

Skillet Steak with Chimichurri

This protein-packed dish features a juicy steak paired with a vibrant chimichurri sauce.

PREP TIME: 15 MINUTES | COOK TIME: DEPENDING ON DESIRED DONENESS (5-10 MINUTES) | YIELDS: 1 SERVING

INGREDIENTS:

- 6 oz lean cut steak (flank steak, skirt steak, or similar)
- 1 tablespoon olive oil
- Salt and black pepper (to taste)

For the Chimichurri Sauce:

- ¼ cup chopped fresh parsley
- 1 tablespoon chopped fresh oregano (or ½ teaspoon dried)
- 1 tablespoon red onion, finely minced
- 1 garlic clove, minced
- 1 tablespoon olive oil
- 1 tablespoon red wine vinegar (or lemon juice)
- Pinch of red pepper flakes (optional)

COOKING INSTRUCTIONS:

1. Make the Chimichurri: In a small bowl, combine chopped parsley, oregano, red onion, garlic, olive oil, red wine vinegar, and red pepper flakes (if using). Stir well and set aside.
2. Prepare the Steak: Pat the steak dry with paper towels. Season generously with salt and pepper on both sides.
3. Heat a grill pan or skillet over medium-high heat. Once hot, sear the steak for 2-3 minutes per side for medium-rare, or adjust time according to your desired doneness.
4. Let the steak rest for 5 minutes before slicing.
5. Serve the sliced steak with a generous spoonful of chimichurri sauce.

NUTRITIONAL INFORMATION: (APPROXIMATE VALUES PER SERVING)

Calories: 450

Phosphorus: 200mg

Protein: 40 grams

Sodium: 60mg (depending on added salt)

Potassium: 100mg (depending on cut of steak)

TIPS FOR MODIFICATION:

- Lean Protein Choice: Select a lean cut of steak to minimize fat content.
- Monitor Sodium Intake: Be mindful of added salt when seasoning the steak.

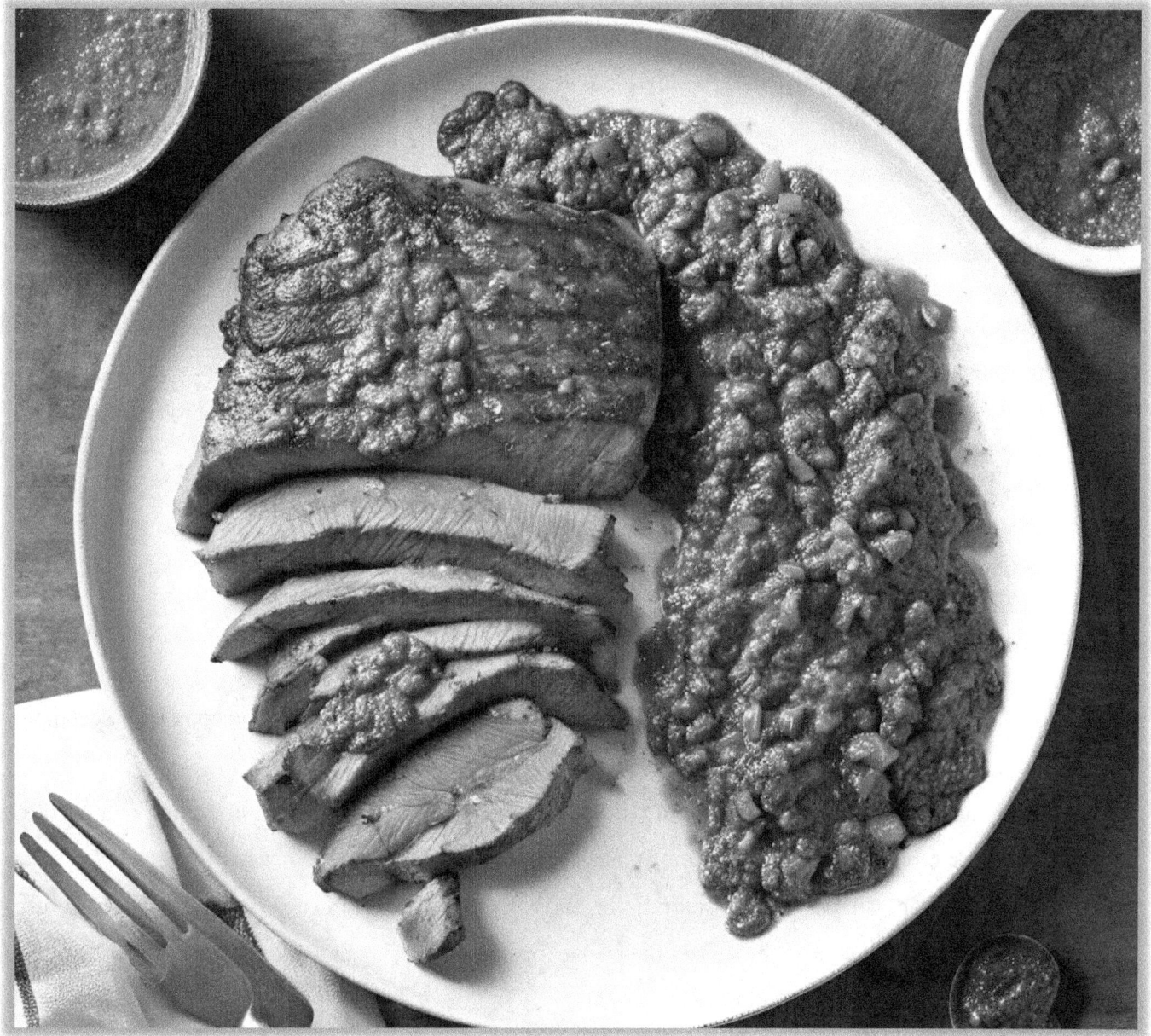

Stuffed Pork Chops with Spinach and Feta

Craving a flavorful and satisfying main course? Look no further than these Stuffed Pork Chops with Spinach and Feta! This recipe is packed with protein and features a delicious spinach and feta cheese filling, making it a perfect CKD-friendly option.

PREP TIME: 15 MINUTES | COOK TIME: 20-25 MINUTES | YIELDS: 2 SERVINGS

INGREDIENTS:

- 2 bone-in pork chops (about 1 inch thick)
- 1 tablespoon olive oil
- Salt and black pepper (to taste)

For the Spinach Feta Filling:

- 2 cups fresh spinach, chopped
- 2 tablespoons crumbled feta cheese
- 1 tablespoon chopped red onion
- 1 garlic clove, minced
- Pinch of dried oregano
- Pinch of red pepper flakes (optional)

COOKING INSTRUCTIONS:

1. Prepare the Filling: In a pan, heat olive oil over medium heat. Add red onion and cook until softened. Add garlic and cook for another minute.
2. Stir in chopped spinach and cook until wilted. Remove from heat and stir in crumbled feta cheese, oregano, and red pepper flakes (if using). Season with salt and pepper to taste.
3. Prepare the Pork Chops: Using a sharp knife, carefully cut a pocket in each pork chop, making sure not to cut all the way through. Season the pork chops generously with salt and pepper on both sides.

4. Stuff each pork chop pocket with the spinach feta mixture. Secure the opening with toothpicks (optional).
5. Heat a skillet over medium heat. Sear the pork chops for 2-3 minutes per side. Reduce heat to medium-low and cook for an additional 15-20 minutes, or until the pork chops are cooked through and the internal temperature reaches 145°F (63°C).
6. Let the pork chops rest for 5 minutes before serving.

NUTRITIONAL INFORMATION: (APPROXIMATE VALUES PER SERVING)

Calories: 400

Phosphorus: 300mg

Protein: 40 grams

Sodium: 100mg (depending on added salt)

Potassium: 250mg (depending on ingredients)

TIPS FOR MODIFICATION:

- Portion Control: Enjoy one stuffed pork chop per serving to manage protein intake.
- Feta Cheese Alternative: Consider a lower-potassium cheese option like mozzarella if needed.

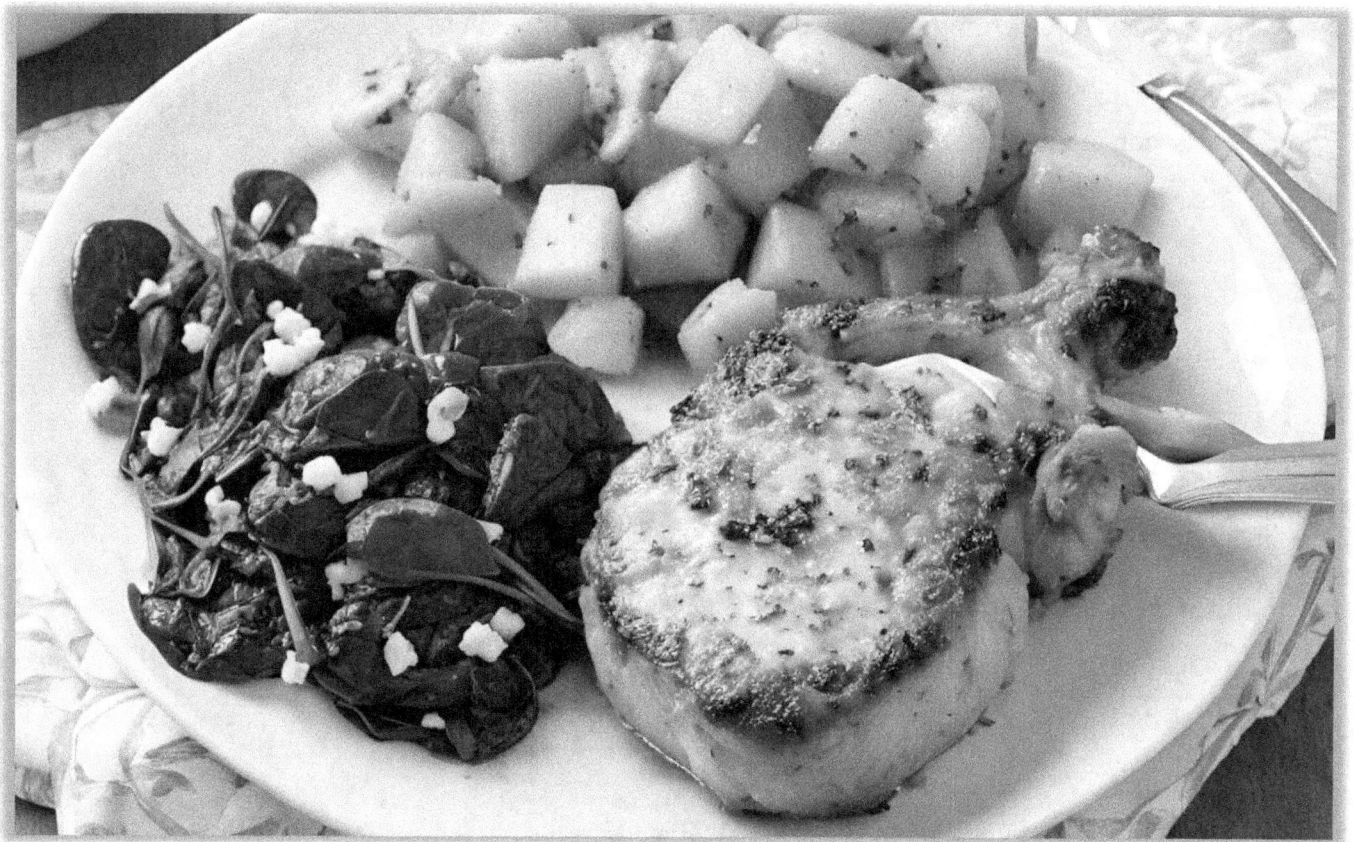

Ground Turkey Meatloaf with Zucchini Noodles

This recipe offers a satisfying twist on a classic comfort food! Made with ground turkey, vegetables, and flavorful spices, this Ground Turkey Meatloaf with Zucchini Noodles is a perfect CKD-friendly main course that's both nutritious and delicious.

PREP TIME: 15 MINUTES | COOK TIME: 45-50 MINUTES | YIELDS: 4 SERVINGS

INGREDIENTS:

- 1 pound ground turkey (90% lean or higher)
- ½ cup chopped onion
- ½ cup grated zucchini (water squeezed out)
- ¼ cup chopped fresh parsley
- 1 large egg, beaten
- ½ cup panko breadcrumbs (or almond flour for lower carb option)
- 1 tablespoon olive oil
- 1 teaspoon dried oregano
- ½ teaspoon garlic powder
- Salt and black pepper (to taste)

For the Zucchini Noodles (Optional):

- 1 medium zucchini, spiralized

COOKING INSTRUCTIONS:

1. Preheat oven to 375°F (190°C). Line a baking sheet with parchment paper.
2. In a large bowl, combine ground turkey, onion, grated zucchini, parsley, beaten egg, panko breadcrumbs (or almond flour), olive oil, oregano, garlic powder, salt, and pepper. Mix well until combined.
3. Form the mixture into a loaf shape on the prepared baking sheet.

4. Optional Zucchini Noodles: If using, spiralize the zucchini and place them around the base of the meatloaf on the baking sheet.
5. Bake the meatloaf for 45-50 minutes, or until the internal temperature reaches 165°F (74°C). Baste the meatloaf occasionally with pan drippings for extra flavor.
6. Let the meatloaf rest for 10 minutes before slicing and serving.

NUTRITIONAL INFORMATION: (APPROXIMATE VALUES PER SERVING)

Calories: 350

Phosphorus: 250mg

Protein: 30 grams

Sodium: 300mg (depending on added salt)

Potassium: 200mg (depending on ingredients)

TIPS FOR MODIFICATION:

- Panko Breadcrumbs: Choose a low-carb option like almond flour or skip the breadcrumbs altogether for a more keto-friendly approach.
- Zucchini Noodles: Consider portion size or omit them entirely if managing carbohydrate intake.

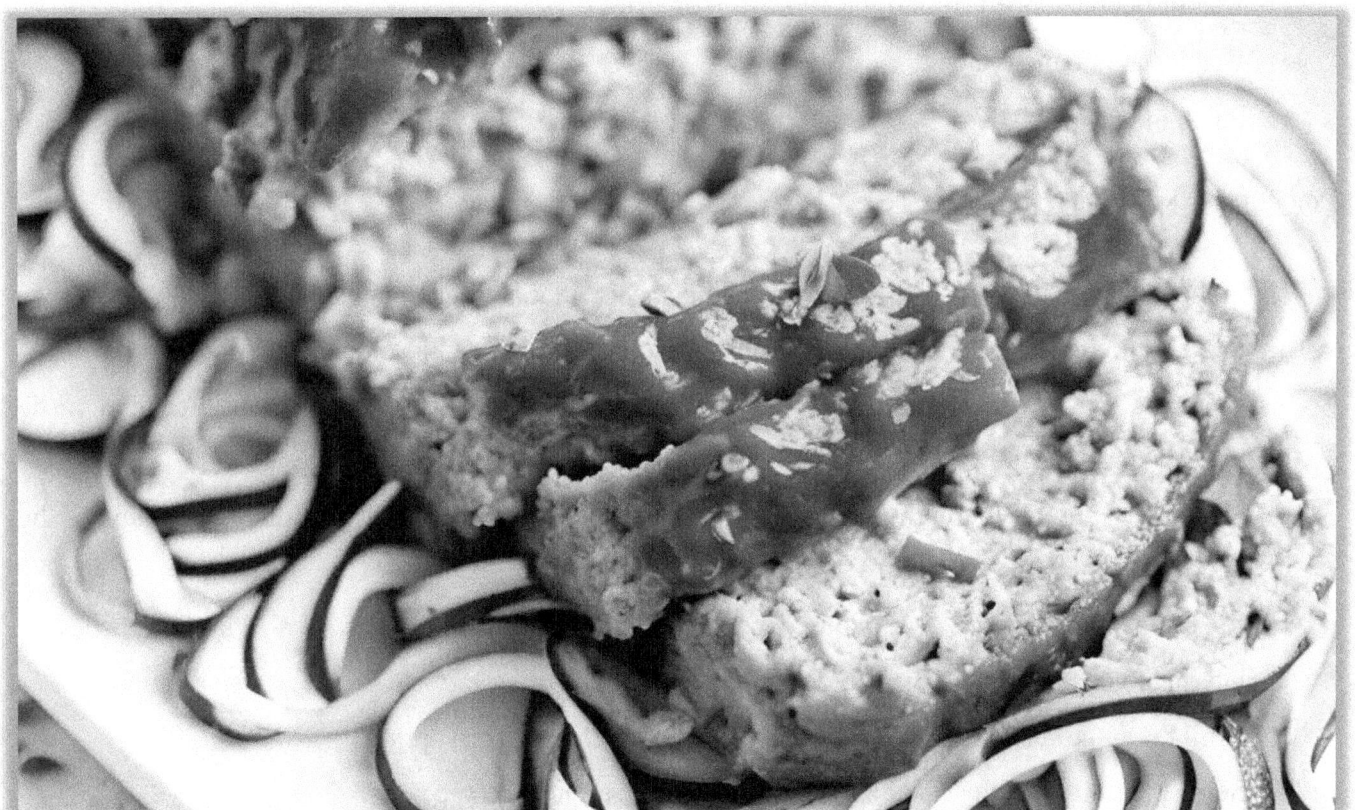

Beef and Broccoli Stir-Fry

This Baked Salmon with Lemon Dill Sauce offers a delicious and healthy main course option! Packed with protein and omega-3 fatty acids, salmon is a perfect choice for a CKD-friendly meal. The light lemon dill sauce adds a burst of flavor without compromising on dietary needs.

PREP TIME: 10 MINUTES | COOK TIME: 12-15 MINUTES | YIELDS: 1 SERVING

INGREDIENTS:

- 6 oz salmon fillet (skin-on or skinless)
- 1 tablespoon olive oil
- Salt and black pepper (to taste)

For the Lemon Dill Sauce:

- 2 tablespoons plain Greek yogurt
- 1 tablespoon mayonnaise (or low-fat option)
- 1 tablespoon chopped fresh dill (or ½ teaspoon dried)
- 1 tablespoon lemon juice
- Pinch of garlic powder

COOKING INSTRUCTIONS:

1. Preheat oven to 400°F (204°C). Line a baking sheet with parchment paper.
2. Pat the salmon fillet dry with paper towels. Season generously with salt and pepper on both sides.
3. In a small bowl, whisk together Greek yogurt, mayonnaise, chopped dill, lemon juice, and garlic powder for the lemon dill sauce.
4. Place the salmon fillet on the prepared baking sheet. Brush the top of the salmon with some of the lemon dill sauce.
5. Bake the salmon for 12-15 minutes, or until the salmon flakes easily with a fork and reaches an internal temperature of 145°F (63°C).
6. Broil the salmon for an additional 1-2 minutes for a crispier top (optional).
7. Serve the salmon with remaining lemon dill sauce spooned on top.

NUTRITIONAL INFORMATION: (APPROXIMATE VALUES PER SERVING)

Calories: 400

Phosphorus: 200mg

Protein: 40 grams

Sodium: 150mg (depending on added

Potassium: 300mg (depending on cut of salmon)

salt)

TIPS FOR MODIFICATION:

- Portion Control: Enjoy a single serving of salmon to manage protein intake.
- Reduced-Potassium Yogurt Option: Choose a plain, unsweetened yogurt option lower in potassium.

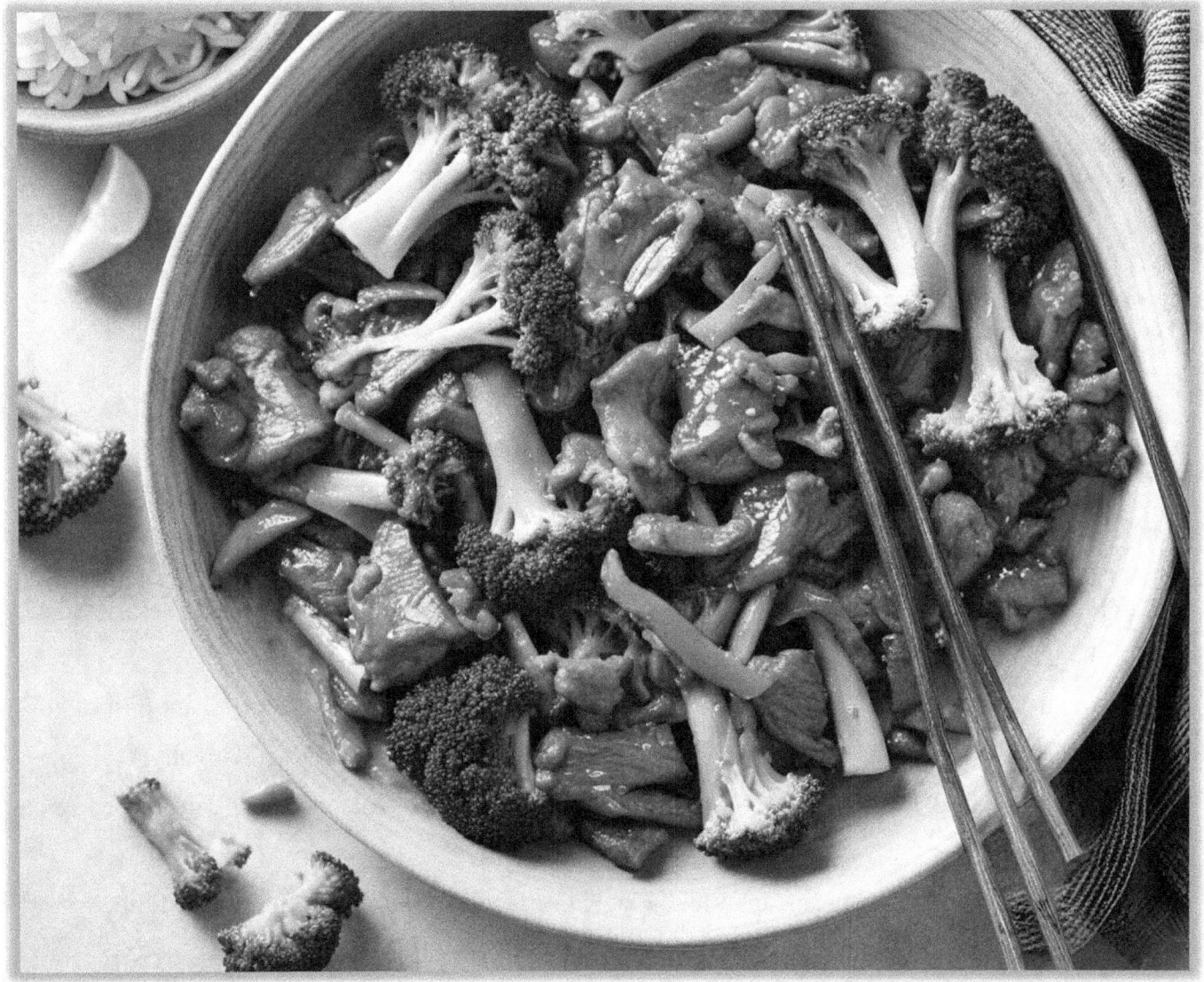

Cod with Tomato Caper Sauce

This recipe is a perfect CKD-friendly option, featuring seared cod fillets bathed in a vibrant tomato sauce with capers and olives.

PREP TIME: 10 MINUTES | COOK TIME: 15-20 MINUTES | YIELDS: 1 SERVING

INGREDIENTS:

- 6 oz cod fillet
- 1 tablespoon olive oil
- Salt and black pepper (to taste)

For the Tomato Caper Sauce:

- 1 tablespoon olive oil
- ¼ cup chopped onion
- 1 clove garlic, minced
- 1 (14.5 oz) can diced tomatoes, drained
- 1 tablespoon capers, drained (rinsed if salt-packed)
- 2 Kalamata olives, chopped (optional)
- Pinch of dried oregano
- Pinch of red pepper flakes (optional)

COOKING INSTRUCTIONS:

1. Make the Sauce: In a saucepan, heat olive oil over medium heat. Add onion and cook until softened, about 3 minutes. Stir in garlic and cook for another minute.
2. Add diced tomatoes, capers, olives (if using), oregano, and red pepper flakes (if using). Bring to a simmer and cook for 5-7 minutes, stirring occasionally, until the sauce thickens slightly.
3. Prepare the Cod: Pat the cod fillet dry with paper towels. Season generously with salt and pepper on both sides.
4. Heat a separate skillet over medium-high heat with 1 tablespoon olive oil. Sear the cod fillet for 3-4 minutes per side, or until cooked through and flakes easily with a fork.

5. Assemble and Serve: Plate the cod fillet and spoon the tomato caper sauce over the top.

NUTRITIONAL INFORMATION: (APPROXIMATE VALUES PER SERVING)

Calories: 350

Phosphorus: 300mg

Protein: 40 grams

Sodium: 200mg (depending on added salt*)*

Potassium: 300mg (depending on ingredients)

TIPS FOR MODIFICATION:

- Monitor Portion Size: Enjoy a single cod fillet to manage protein intake.
- Lower-Potassium Tomato Option: Choose cherry tomatoes or a diced tomato option labeled "potassium-reduced" if available.

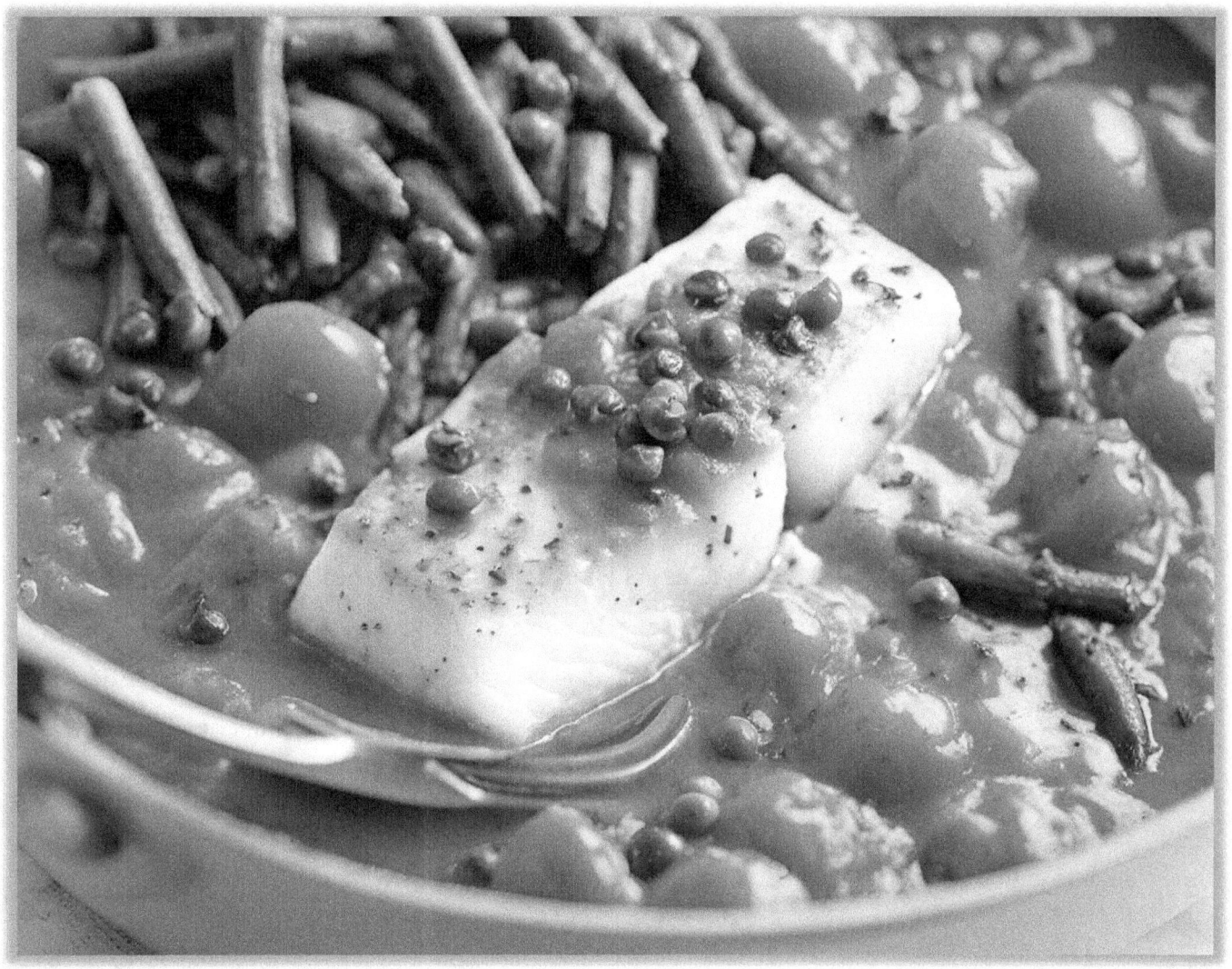

Shrimp Scampi with Zucchini Noodles

Enjoy the flavors of classic Shrimp Scampi in a CKD-friendly way! This recipe features succulent shrimp tossed in a garlicky lemon sauce, served over refreshing zucchini noodles for a satisfying and lower-carb main course.

PREP TIME: 10 MINUTES | COOK TIME: 10-12 MINUTES | YIELDS: 1 SERVING

INGREDIENTS:

- 5 oz shrimp, peeled and deveined
- 1 tablespoon olive oil
- 2 cloves garlic, minced
- ¼ cup dry white wine (or chicken broth)
- 1 tablespoon lemon juice
- Pinch of red pepper flakes (optional)
- Salt and black pepper (to taste)
- 1 medium zucchini, spiralized (or spaghetti squash noodles for a different option)

COOKING INSTRUCTIONS:

1. Prepare the Zucchini Noodles: Using a spiralizer, create zucchini noodles from the zucchini. Alternatively, prepare spaghetti squash noodles if desired.
2. Cook the Shrimp: Heat olive oil in a large skillet over medium-high heat. Add shrimp and cook for 2-3 minutes per side, or until pink and opaque. Remove shrimp from the pan and set aside.
3. Make the Sauce: In the same skillet, add garlic and cook for 30 seconds, until fragrant. Add white wine (or broth), lemon juice, and red pepper flakes (if using). Bring to a simmer and cook for 2-3 minutes, or until slightly reduced. Season with salt and pepper to taste.
4. Assemble and Serve: Toss the cooked shrimp back into the pan with the sauce. Heat for another minute until warmed through. Serve immediately over the prepared zucchini noodles.

NUTRITIONAL INFORMATION: (APPROXIMATE VALUES PER SERVING)

Calories: 300

Phosphorus: 350mg

Protein: 30 grams

Sodium: 100mg (depending on added

Potassium: 250mg (depending on ingredients)

salt)

TIPS FOR MODIFICATION:

- Portion Control: Enjoy a single serving of shrimp to manage protein intake.
- Vegetable Option: Consider using spaghetti squash noodles for a slightly higher carbohydrate option if needed for CKD management.

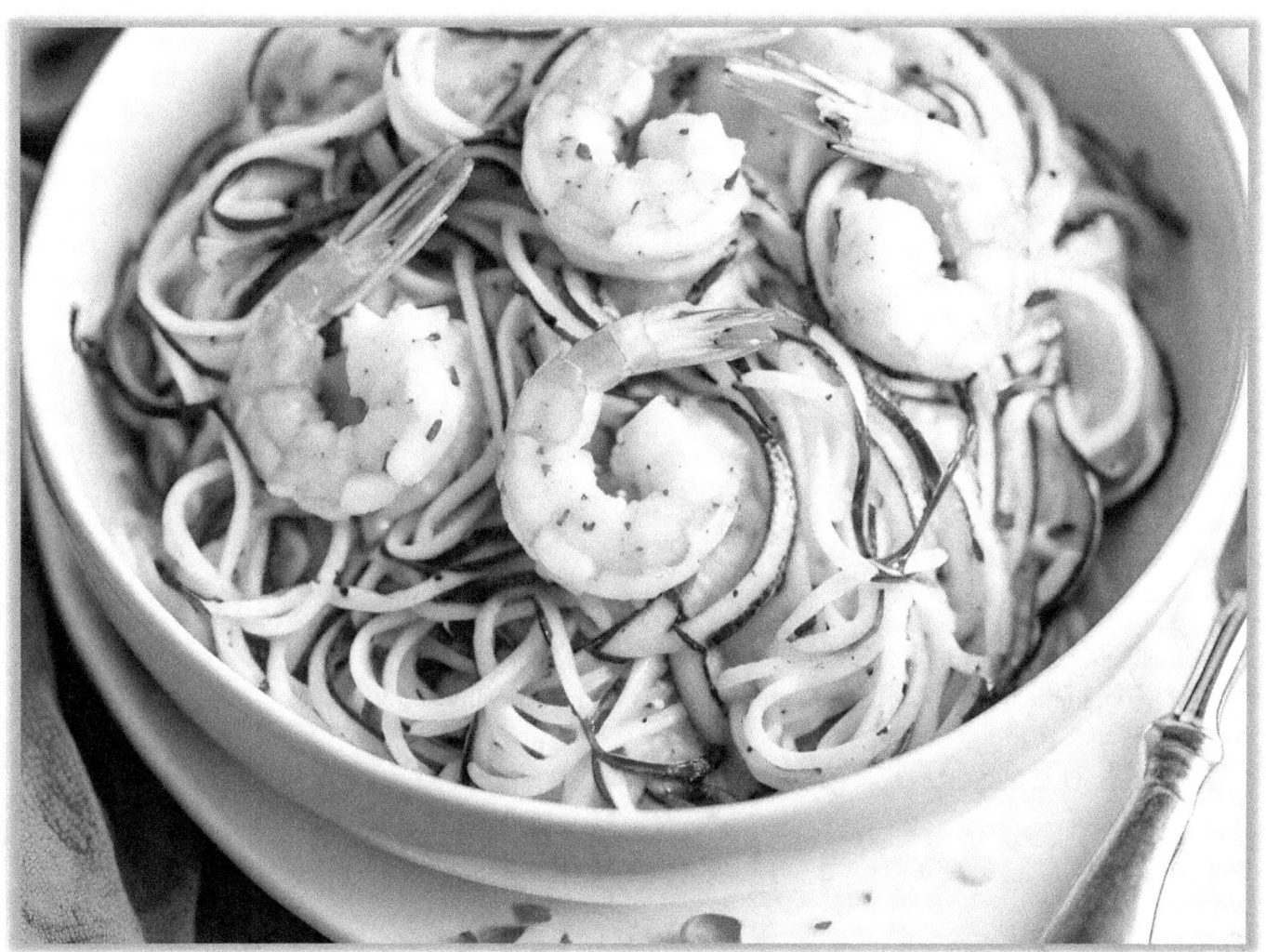

Tuna Salad with Celery and Avocado

This Tuna Salad with Celery and Avocado offers a light and flavorful main course option perfect for busy days! Packed with protein and healthy fats, it's a delicious and convenient choice for a CKD-friendly meal.

PREP TIME: 10 MINUTES | COOK TIME: NO COOK TIME | YIELDS: 1 SERVING

INGREDIENTS:

- 5 oz canned tuna in water, drained
- ½ cup chopped celery
- ½ avocado, mashed
- 1 tablespoon mayonnaise (or low-fat option)
- 1 tablespoon lemon juice
- Salt and black pepper (to taste)

Optional Add-Ins:

- Chopped red onion
- Fresh herbs (parsley, dill)

COOKING INSTRUCTIONS:

1. In a bowl, combine flaked tuna, chopped celery, mashed avocado, mayonnaise, lemon juice, salt, and pepper.
2. Gently fold in any optional add-ins like red onion or fresh herbs.
3. Serve immediately on a bed of lettuce or enjoy wrapped in low-carb tortillas.

NUTRITIONAL INFORMATION: (APPROXIMATE VALUES PER SERVING)

Calories: 350

Potassium: 300mg (depending on ingredients)

Protein: 30 grams

Phosphorus: 200mg

Sodium: 150mg (depending on added salt)

TIPS FOR MODIFICATION:

- Mayonnaise Choice: Opt for a low-fat or light mayonnaise to reduce fat content.
- Portion Control: Enjoy a single serving of tuna salad to manage protein intake.

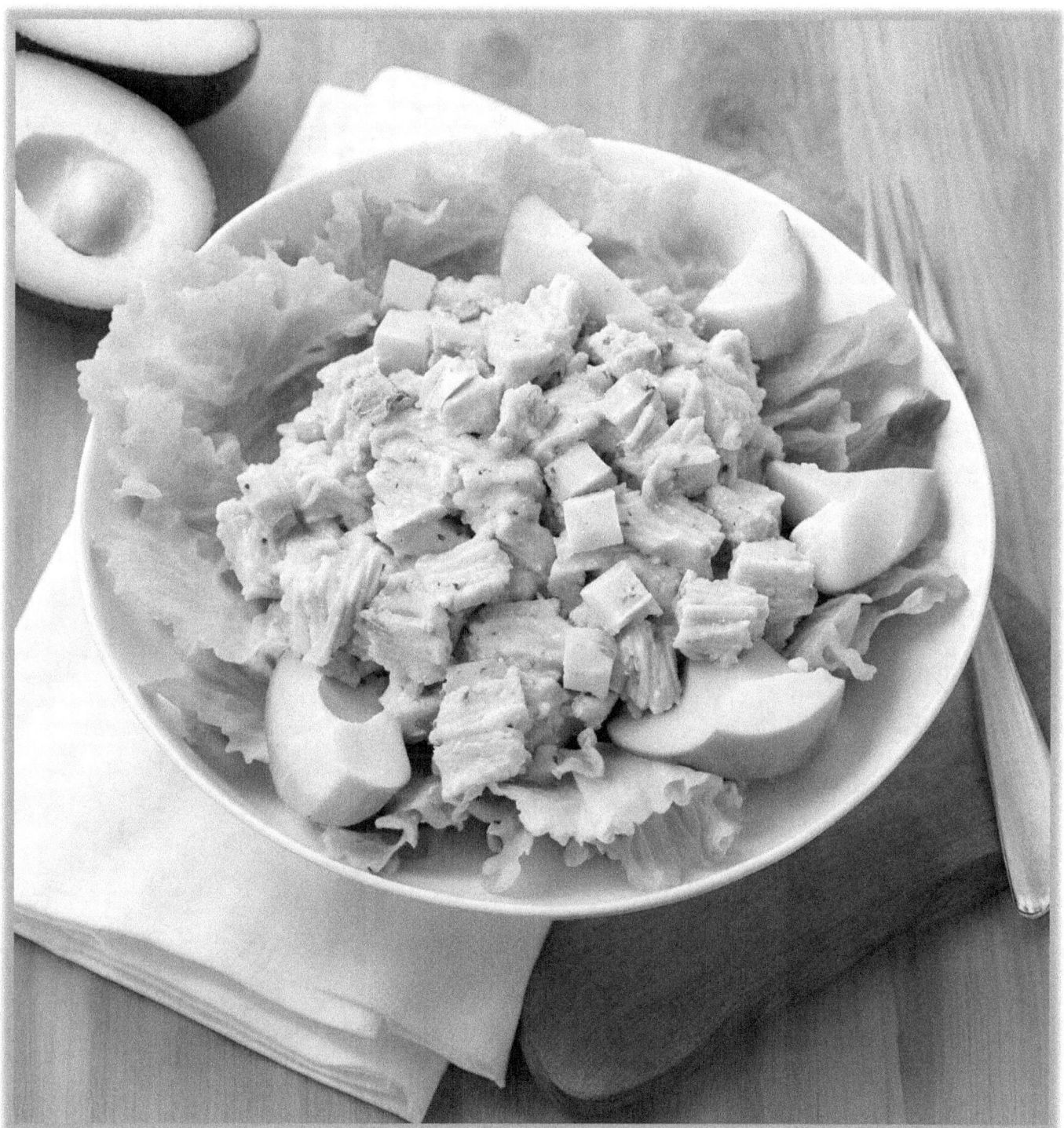

Blackened Tilapia with Cajun Seasoning

Spice up your dinner routine with Blackened Tilapia with Cajun Seasoning! This dish is packed with bold flavors and protein, making it a perfect CKD-friendly main course option.

PREP TIME: 10 MINUTES | COOK TIME: 4-5 MINUTES PER SIDE | YIELDS: 1 SERVING

INGREDIENTS:

- 6 oz tilapia fillet
- 1 tablespoon olive oil
- 2 tablespoons Cajun seasoning

COOKING INSTRUCTIONS:

1. Pat the tilapia fillet dry with paper towels. Season generously with Cajun seasoning on both sides.
2. Heat olive oil in a large skillet over medium-high heat. Once hot, carefully place the seasoned tilapia fillet in the pan.
3. Sear the tilapia for 4-5 minutes per side, or until cooked through and flakes easily with a fork. The blackened seasoning will create a dark, flavorful crust.

NUTRITIONAL INFORMATION: (APPROXIMATE VALUES PER SERVING)

Calories: 300

Protein: 40 grams

Potassium: 350mg (depending on brand of Cajun seasoning)

Phosphorus: 200mg

Sodium: 200mg (depending on added salt)

TIPS FOR MODIFICATION:

- Monitor Potassium: Cajun seasoning can vary in potassium content. Choose a low-sodium option if managing potassium intake.
- Portion Control: Enjoy a single serving of tilapia to manage protein intake.

Baked Salmon with Lemon Dill Sauce

This recipe offers a light and flavorful main course perfect for busy weeknights! Packed with protein and omega-3 fatty acids, salmon is a great choice for a CKD-friendly meal. The easy lemon dill sauce adds a burst of brightness without compromising on dietary needs.

PREP TIME: 10 MINUTES | COOK TIME: 12-15 MINUTES | YIELDS: 1 SERVING

INGREDIENTS:

- 6 oz salmon fillet (skin-on or skinless)
- 1 tablespoon olive oil
- Salt and black pepper (to taste)

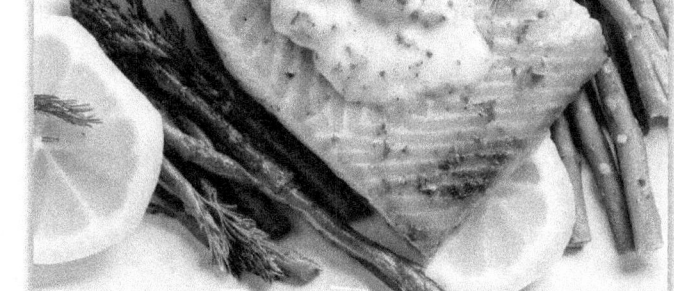

For the Lemon Dill Sauce:

- 2 tablespoons plain Greek yogurt (or sour cream for a richer option)
- 1 tablespoon mayonnaise (or low-fat option)
- 1 tablespoon chopped fresh dill (or ½ teaspoon dried)
- 1 tablespoon lemon juice
- Pinch of garlic powder

COOKING INSTRUCTIONS:

1. Preheat oven to 400°F (204°C). Line a baking sheet with parchment paper.
2. Pat the salmon fillet dry with paper towels. Season generously with salt and pepper on both sides.
3. In a small bowl, whisk together Greek yogurt (or sour cream), mayonnaise, chopped dill, lemon juice, and garlic powder for the lemon dill sauce.
4. Place the salmon fillet on the prepared baking sheet. Brush the top of the salmon with some of the lemon dill sauce.
5. Bake the salmon for 12-15 minutes, or until the salmon flakes easily with a fork and reaches an internal temperature of 145°F (63°C).

6. Broil the salmon for an additional 1-2 minutes for a crispier top (optional).
7. Serve the salmon with remaining lemon dill sauce spooned on top.

NUTRITIONAL INFORMATION: (APPROXIMATE VALUES PER SERVING)

Calories: 400

Phosphorus: 200mg

Protein: 40 grams

Sodium: 150mg (depending on added salt)

Potassium: 300mg (depending on cut of salmon)

TIPS FOR MODIFICATION:

- Portion Control: Enjoy a single serving of salmon to manage protein intake.
- Reduced-Potassium Yogurt Option: Choose a plain, unsweetened yogurt option lower in potassium.

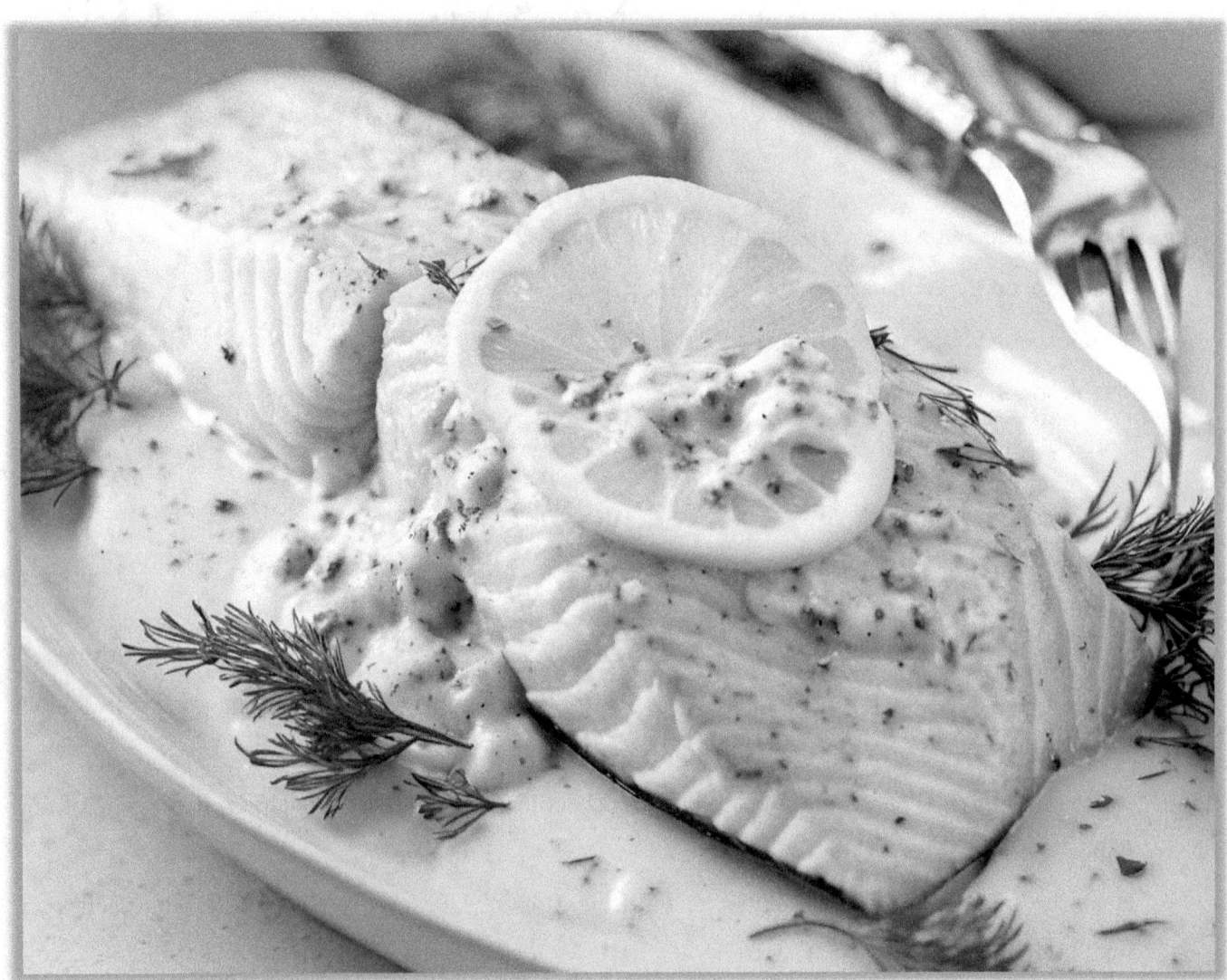

SOUPS AND SALADS

Chicken and Vegetable Soup

Warm up with a hearty and satisfying Chicken and Vegetable Soup! This comforting recipe is a perfect CKD-friendly main course option, packed with protein and flavorful vegetables.

PREP TIME: 10 MINUTES | COOK TIME: 30-40 MINUTES | YIELDS: 4 SERVINGS

INGREDIENTS:

- 1 tablespoon olive oil
- 1 onion, chopped
- 2 carrots, diced
- 2 celery stalks, diced
- 4 cloves garlic, minced
- 4 cups low-sodium chicken broth
- 4 cups water
- 1-pound boneless, skinless chicken breasts, chopped
- 1 cup chopped low-potassium vegetables (broccoli florets, green beans, mushrooms)
- ½ teaspoon dried thyme
- ½ teaspoon dried parsley
- Salt and black pepper (to taste)

Optional Ingredients:

- Cooked rice or quinoa (for a more substantial meal, consider a small portion)
- Chopped fresh herbs (parsley, dill) for garnish

COOKING INSTRUCTIONS:

1. Heat olive oil in a large pot over medium heat. Add onion, carrots, and celery. Cook until softened, about 5 minutes.

2. Stir in garlic and cook for an additional minute.
3. Pour in chicken broth and water. Bring to a boil.
4. Add chopped chicken breasts, thyme, and parsley. Reduce heat and simmer for 15-20 minutes, or until chicken is cooked through.
5. Stir in chopped low-potassium vegetables and cook for an additional 5-7 minutes, or until tender-crisp.
6. Season with salt and pepper to taste.

NUTRITIONAL INFORMATION: (APPROXIMATE VALUES PER SERVING)

Calories: 300

Phosphorus: 250mg

Protein: 30 grams

Sodium: 100mg (depending on added salt)

Potassium: 350mg (depending on vegetables used)

TIPS FOR MODIFICATION:

- Vegetable Selection: Choose low-potassium vegetables like broccoli florets, green beans, or mushrooms.
- Rice or Quinoa (Optional): If adding rice or quinoa, use a small portion to manage carbohydrate intake.

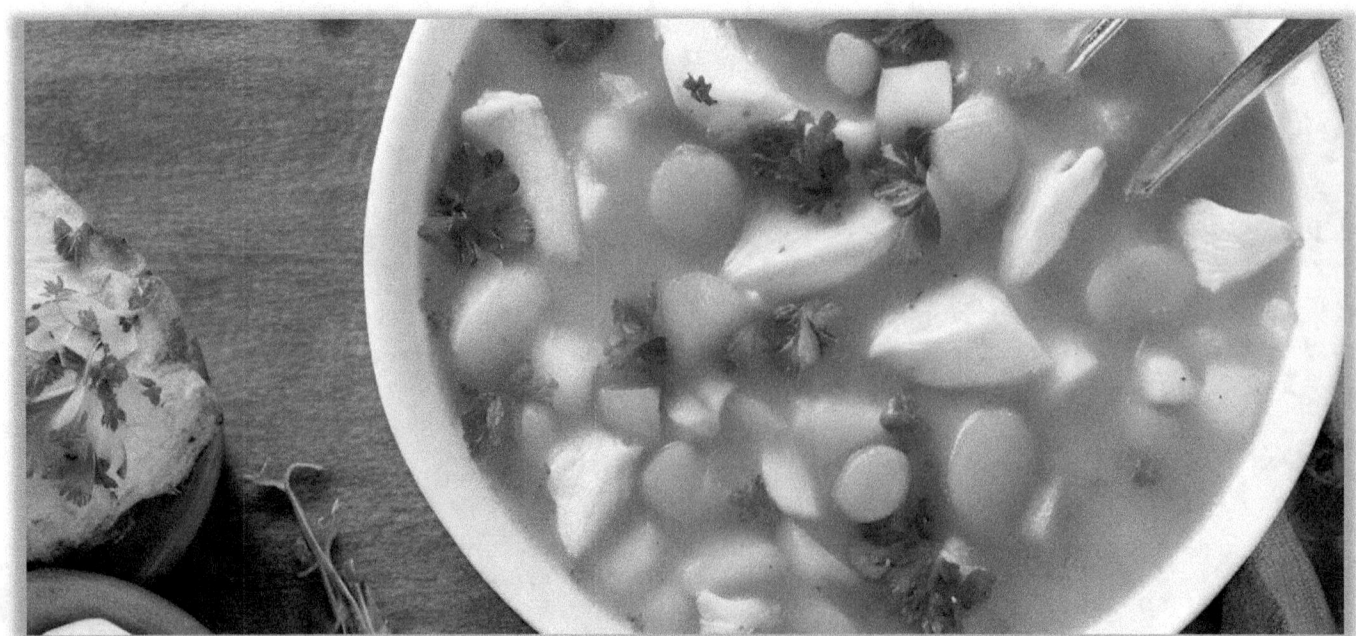

Creamy Keto Cauliflower Soup

This Creamy Keto Cauliflower Soup is your answer! Packed with roasted cauliflower and a rich, flavorful broth, it's a satisfying CKD-friendly main course that's both delicious and low-carb.

PREP TIME: 10 MINUTES | COOK TIME: 30 MINUTES | YIELDS: 4 SERVINGS

INGREDIENTS:

- 1 head cauliflower, roughly chopped
- 1 tablespoon olive oil
- 1 onion, diced
- 4 cloves garlic, minced
- 4 cups chicken broth
- 1 cup unsweetened almond milk (or low-carb dairy alternative)
- 4 oz cream cheese, softened (or full-fat ricotta cheese for a tangier option)
- ½ teaspoon dried thyme
- Salt and black pepper (to taste)

Optional Toppings:

- Chopped fresh chives
- Shredded cheddar cheese (small amount for a richer flavor)

COOKING INSTRUCTIONS:

1. Preheat oven to 400°F (204°C). Toss cauliflower florets with olive oil and spread on a baking sheet. Roast for 20-25 minutes, or until tender-crisp.
2. While cauliflower roasts, heat remaining olive oil in a large pot over medium heat. Add onion and garlic, cook until softened, about 5 minutes.
3. Pour in chicken broth and bring to a simmer. Add roasted cauliflower florets and simmer for an additional 5 minutes.
4. Using an immersion blender or transferring batches to a blender, puree the soup until smooth. Alternatively, leave the soup with a chunky texture if desired.

5. Stir in unsweetened almond milk, cream cheese (or ricotta cheese), and thyme. Heat gently until cream cheese melts and soup is heated through.
6. Season with salt and pepper to taste.

NUTRITIONAL INFORMATION: (APPROXIMATE VALUES PER SERVING)

Calories: 350

Phosphorus: 300mg

Protein: 20 grams

Sodium: 150mg (depending on added salt)

Potassium: 250mg (depending on ingredients)

TIPS FOR CKD MODIFICATION:

- Dairy Choice: Opt for unsweetened almond milk or a low-carb dairy alternative to manage carbohydrate intake.
- Cheese Topping (Optional): Enjoy a small amount of shredded cheese for added flavor, keeping in mind its impact on protein and fat intake.

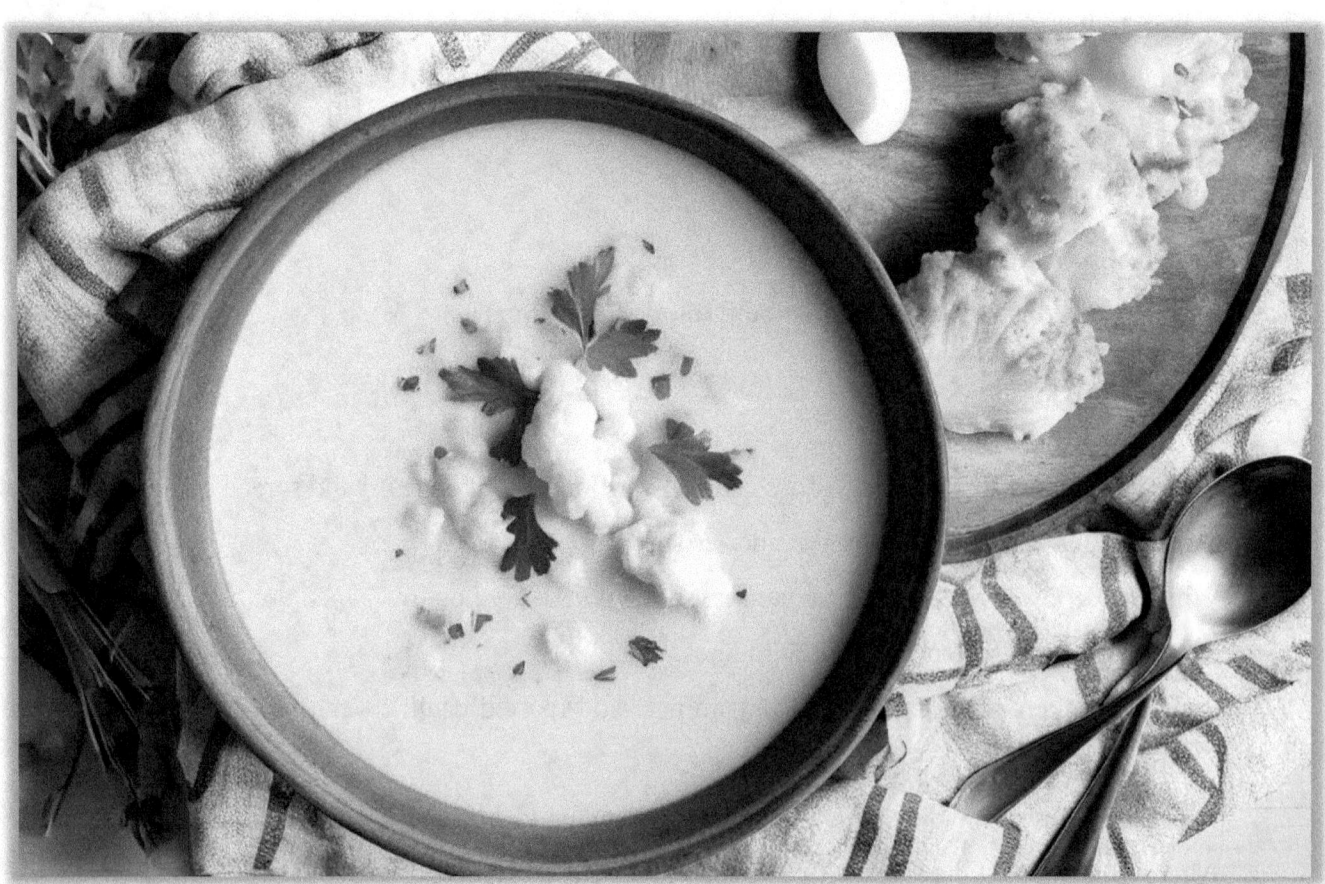

Taco Soup with Ground Beef

This Taco Soup with Ground Beef is a hearty CKD-friendly main course option, packed with protein and all your favorite taco fixings.

PREP TIME: 10 MINUTES | COOK TIME: 20-25 MINUTES | YIELDS: 4 SERVINGS

INGREDIENTS:

- 1 tablespoon olive oil
- 1 pound ground beef (90% lean or higher)
- 1 onion, chopped
- 1 green bell pepper, diced (optional)
- 1 (15 oz) can diced tomatoes, undrained
- 1 (15.25 oz) can low-sodium kidney beans, drained and rinsed
- 1 (15 oz) can black beans, drained and rinsed
- 1 (14.5 oz) can diced tomatoes with green chilies (Rotel or similar), undrained (optional)
- 4 cups low-sodium chicken broth
- 1 tablespoon taco seasoning
- 1 teaspoon chili powder (optional)
- Salt and black pepper (to taste)

<u>**Optional Toppings:**</u>

- Shredded cheese (small amount)
- Chopped avocado
- Sour cream
- Cilantro

COOKING INSTRUCTIONS:

1. Heat olive oil in a large pot or Dutch oven over medium heat. Add ground beef and cook until browned, breaking it up with a spoon.

2. Stir in onion and green pepper (if using). Cook until softened, about 5 minutes.
3. Add diced tomatoes (with or without chilies), kidney beans, black beans, chicken broth, taco seasoning, and chili powder (if using). Bring to a boil, then reduce heat and simmer for 15-20 minutes, or until flavors meld.
4. Season with salt and pepper to taste.

NUTRITIONAL INFORMATION: (APPROXIMATE VALUES PER SERVING)

Calories: 400

Phosphorus: 300mg

Protein: 40 grams

Sodium: 300mg (depending on added salt)

Potassium: 500mg (depending on ingredients)

TIPS FOR MODIFICATION:

- Portion Control: Enjoy a single serving of soup to manage protein and carbohydrate intake.
- Toppings: Opt for a small amount of cheese or skip it altogether. Consider using avocado or chopped low-carb vegetables for toppings.

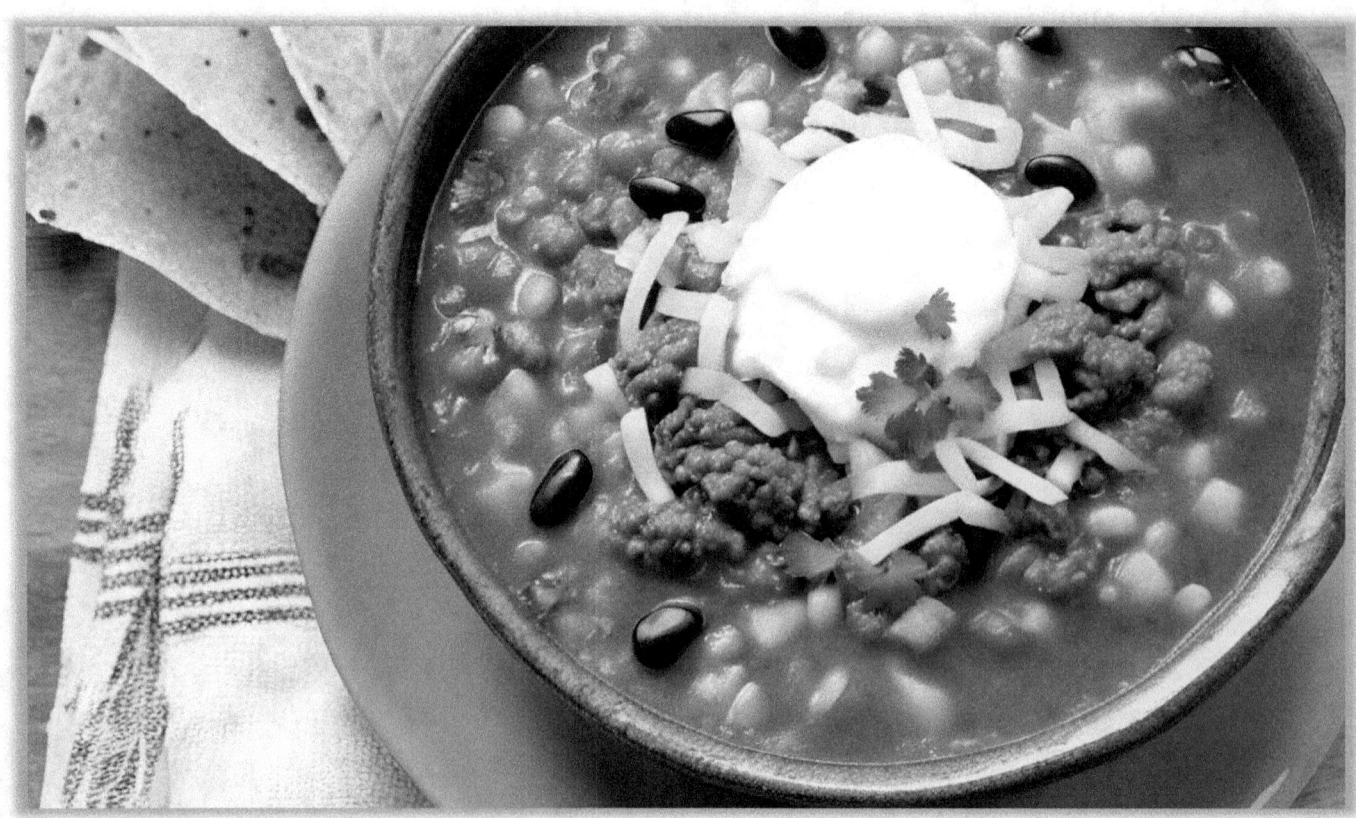

Italian Wedding Soup with Meatballs

Enjoy a taste of Italy with this comforting Italian Wedding Soup with Meatballs! Packed with protein and tiny pasta balls, it's a familiar favorite transformed into a CKD-friendly main course.

PREP TIME: 15 MINUTES | COOK TIME: 30-35 MINUTES | YIELDS: 2 SERVINGS

INGREDIENTS:

For the Meatballs:

- ¾ lb. ground beef (90% lean or higher)
- ¼ cup grated Parmesan cheese
- 1 tablespoon chopped fresh parsley
- 1 large egg, beaten
- ⅓ cup Italian seasoned bread crumbs (or almond flour for lower carb option)
- Pinch of salt and black pepper

For the Soup:

- 8 cups chicken broth
- 2 cups chopped escarole or spinach
- 1 cup chopped carrots
- ½ cup chopped celery
- ¼ cup small pasta (like pastina or ditalini)
- Salt and black pepper (to taste)

Optional Garnish:

- Grated Parmesan cheese

COOKING INSTRUCTIONS:

1. Make the Meatballs: In a bowl, combine ground beef, Parmesan cheese, parsley, egg, bread crumbs (or almond flour), salt, and pepper. Mix well and form into small, bite-sized meatballs.
2. In a large pot, bring chicken broth to a simmer. Add carrots and celery, cook for 5 minutes.
3. Gently roll the meatballs into the simmering broth. Cook for 10-12 minutes, or until meatballs are cooked through.
4. Stir in chopped escarole or spinach and small pasta. Cook for an additional 2-3 minutes, or until pasta is al dente.
5. Season with salt and pepper to taste.

NUTRITIONAL INFORMATION: (APPROXIMATE VALUES PER SERVING)

Calories: 400

Phosphorus: 350mg

Protein: 40 grams

Sodium: 200mg (depending on added salt)

Potassium: 300mg (depending on ingredients)

TIPS FOR MODIFICATION:

- Pasta Portion: Use a small, measured amount of pasta to manage carbohydrate intake.
- Breadcrumbs: Consider using a low-carb option like almond flour for the meatballs or skipping breadcrumbs altogether.

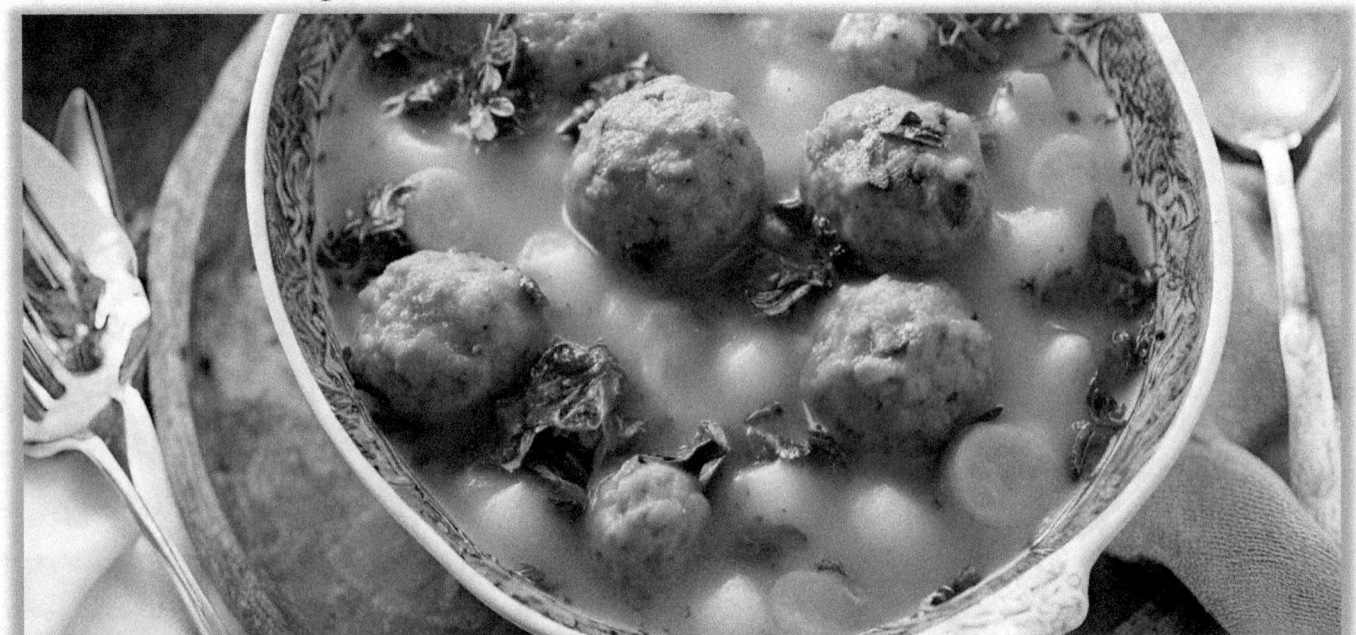

Lentil Soup (moderate portion)

This Lentil Soup is a delicious and satisfying main course option that's easy on the wallet! Packed with protein and fiber-rich lentils, it's a nourishing choice. This recipe is made for a moderate portion size, perfect for those watching calorie intake or following a CKD diet.

PREP TIME: 10 MINUTES | COOK TIME: 30-35 MINUTES | YIELDS: 2 SERVINGS

INGREDIENTS:

- 1 tablespoon olive oil
- 1 onion, chopped
- 2 carrots, diced
- 1 celery stalk, diced
- 2 cloves garlic, minced
- ¾ cup dry green lentils, rinsed
- 4 cups low-sodium vegetable broth
- 1 (14.5 oz) can diced tomatoes, undrained
- ½ teaspoon dried thyme
- Salt and black pepper (to taste)

Optional Ingredients:

- 1 bay leaf
- 1 cup chopped kale or spinach (added in last 5 minutes of cooking)

COOKING INSTRUCTIONS:

1. Heat olive oil in a large pot or Dutch oven over medium heat. Add onion, carrots, and celery. Cook until softened, about 5 minutes.
2. Stir in garlic and cook for an additional minute.
3. Add rinsed lentils, vegetable broth, diced tomatoes, thyme, and bay leaf (if using). Bring to a boil, then reduce heat and simmer for 20-25 minutes, or until lentils are tender.

4. Remove bay leaf (if using) and stir in chopped kale or spinach (if using). Cook for an additional 5 minutes, or until wilted.
5. Season with salt and pepper to taste.

NUTRITIONAL INFORMATION: (APPROXIMATE VALUES PER SERVING)

Calories: 300

Phosphorus: 200mg

Protein: 18 grams

Sodium: 300mg (depending on added salt)

Potassium: 400mg (depending on ingredients)

TIPS FOR MODIFICATION:

- Portion Control: This recipe is already a moderate portion size, suitable for CKD management.
- Vegetable Selection: Choose lower-potassium vegetables like green beans or mushrooms instead of kale or spinach if needed.

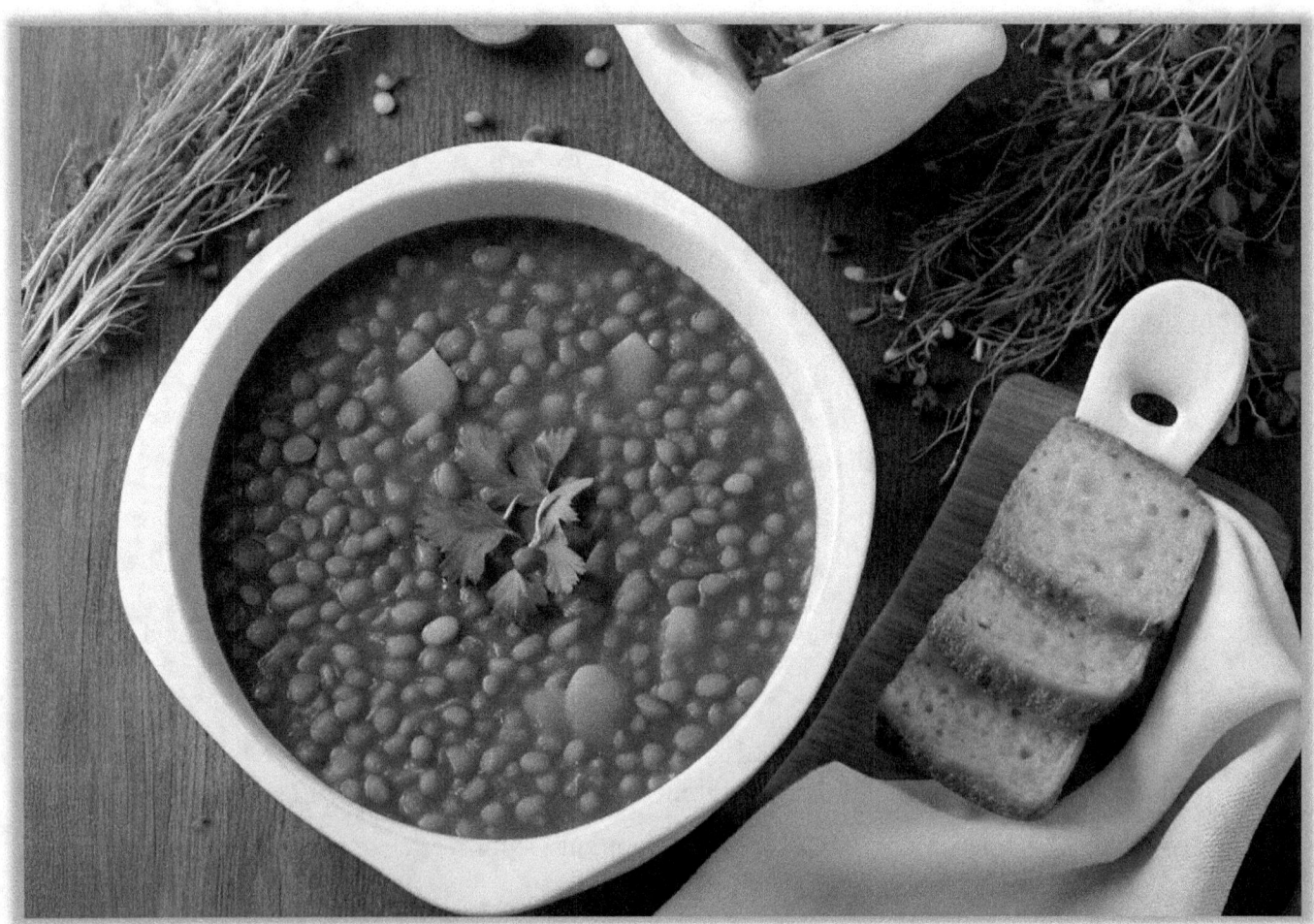

Steak Salad with Blue Cheese and Arugula

This recipe is a perfect marriage of elegance and dietary needs! Packed with protein and healthy fats, it features juicy grilled steak on a bed of peppery arugula and crumbles of tangy blue cheese. Ideal for a satisfying CKD-friendly main course.

PREP TIME: 10 MINUTES | COOK TIME: VARIES DEPENDING ON STEAK THICKNESS | YIELDS: 1 SERVING

INGREDIENTS:

- 6 oz ribeye steak (or preferred cut)
- 1 tablespoon olive oil
- Salt and black pepper (to taste)
- 2 cups baby arugula
- ¼ cup crumbled blue cheese
- 1 tablespoon sliced red onion (optional)
- Cherry tomatoes (optional)
- 2 tablespoons balsamic vinaigrette (or your preferred low-carb dressing)

COOKING INSTRUCTIONS:

1. Prepare the Steak: Pat the steak dry with paper towels. Season generously with salt and pepper on both sides. Heat a grill pan or skillet over medium-high heat. Sear the steak for 3-4 minutes per side for medium-rare, or according to your preference. Let the steak rest for 5 minutes before slicing.
2. Assemble the Salad: In a large bowl, toss arugula with balsamic vinaigrette (or dressing of choice).
3. Plate the dressed arugula, top with sliced steak, crumbled blue cheese, red onion (if using), and cherry tomatoes (if using).

NUTRITIONAL INFORMATION: (APPROXIMATE VALUES PER SERVING)

Calories: 500 *Protein: 40 grams*

Potassium: 200mg (depending on ingredients)   *Sodium: 350mg (depending on added salt)*

Phosphorus: 300mg

TIPS FOR MODIFICATION:

- Portion Control: Enjoy a single serving of steak to manage protein intake.
- Dressing Choice: Opt for a low-carb vinaigrette or dressing to avoid added sugars. Consider a simple olive oil and balsamic vinegar mixture for a classic touch.

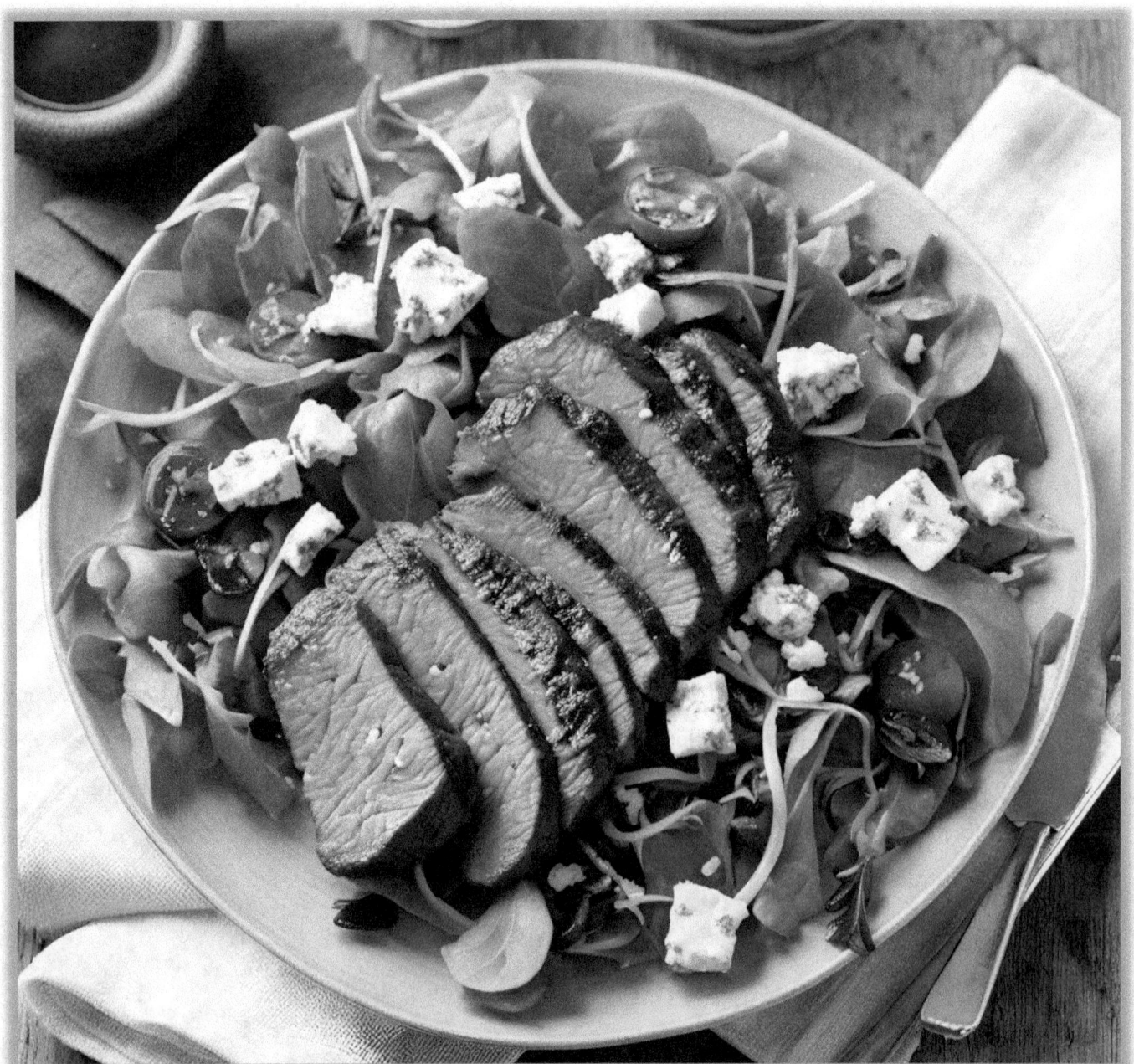

Grilled Chicken Caesar Salad

This recipe features juicy grilled chicken breast on a bed of romaine lettuce with a creamy Caesar dressing, perfect for a satisfying and CKD-friendly main course.

PREP TIME: 15 MINUTES | COOK TIME: 10-12 MINUTES | YIELDS: 1 SERVING

INGREDIENTS:

- 4 oz boneless, skinless chicken breast
- 1 tablespoon olive oil
- Salt and black pepper (to taste)
- 2 cups romaine lettuce, chopped
- 1/4 cup shredded Parmesan cheese
- Caesar Dressing (see recipe below or store-bought low-carb option)

For the Easy Caesar Dressing (Optional):

- 2 tablespoons mayonnaise (or low-fat option)
- 1 tablespoon lemon juice
- 1 anchovy fillet (optional, for umami flavor)
- 1 clove garlic, minced
- 1/4 teaspoon Dijon mustard
- Pinch of dried oregano
- Salt and black pepper (to taste)

COOKING INSTRUCTIONS:

1. Marinate the Chicken (Optional): In a bowl, toss chicken breast with olive oil, salt, and pepper. Marinate for 15 minutes (or up to 30 minutes) for added flavor, if desired.
2. Prepare the Caesar Dressing (Optional): In a small bowl, whisk together mayonnaise, lemon juice, anchovy (if using), garlic, Dijon mustard, oregano, salt, and pepper.
3. Cook the Chicken: Preheat grill pan or skillet over medium-high heat. Grill chicken breast for 5-6 minutes per side, or until cooked through.

4. Assemble the Salad: On a plate, arrange chopped romaine lettuce. Top with sliced grilled chicken, shredded Parmesan cheese, and drizzle with Caesar dressing of choice.

NUTRITIONAL INFORMATION: (APPROXIMATE VALUES PER SERVING)

Calories: 400

Phosphorus: 250mg

Protein: 40 grams

Sodium: 300mg (depending on added salt)

Potassium: 200mg (depending on ingredients)

TIPS FOR MODIFICATION:

- Portion Control: Enjoy a single serving of chicken breast to manage protein intake.
- Dressing Choice: Opt for a low-carb store-bought Caesar dressing or use the homemade version above, skipping the anchovy for a lower sodium option.

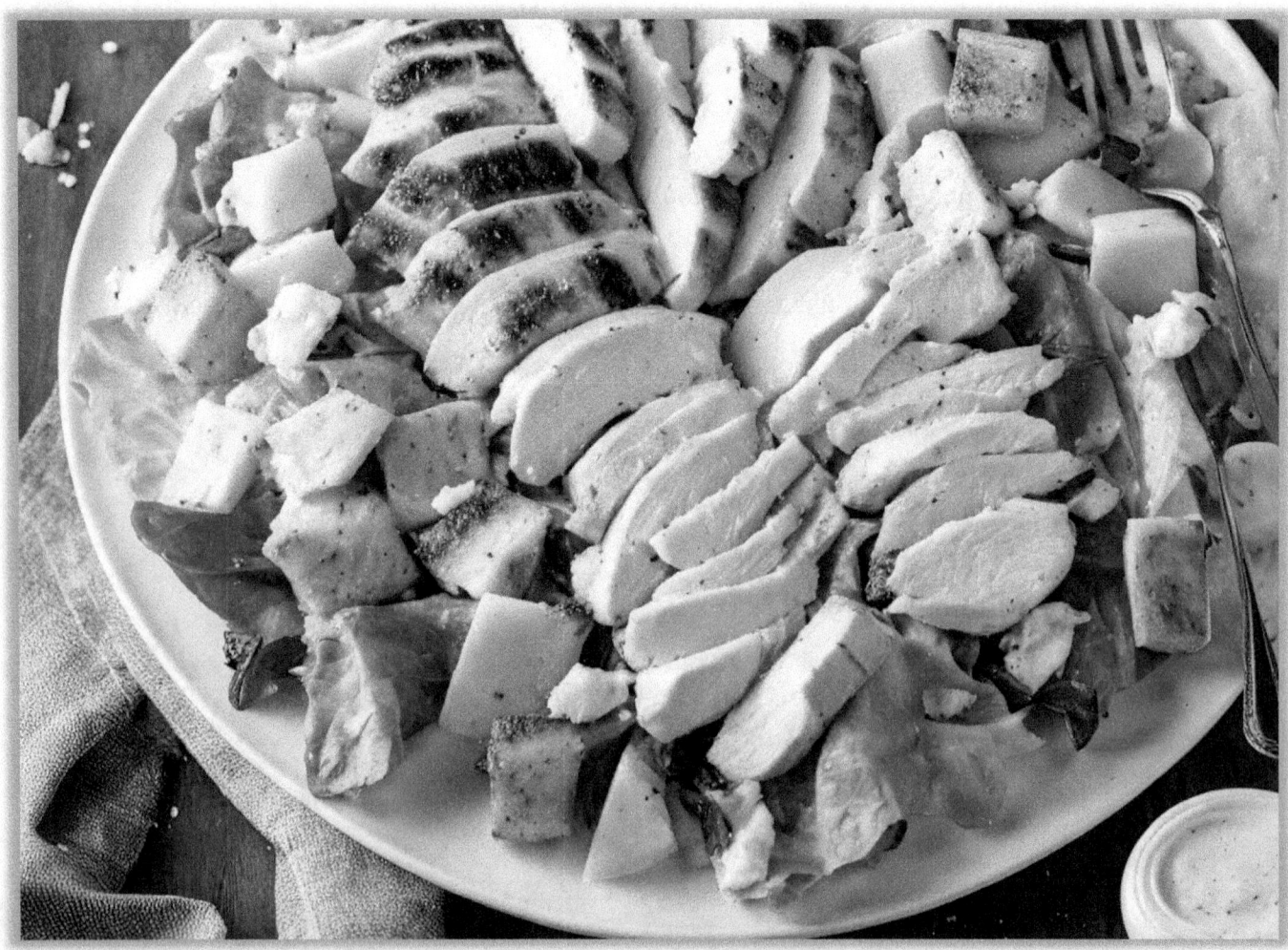

Cobb Salad with Grilled Chicken and Avocado

This recipe is a perfect CKD-friendly main course option, featuring grilled chicken, avocado, and all your favorite salad fixings.

PREP TIME: 15 MINUTES | COOK TIME: 10-12 MINUTES | YIELDS: 1 SERVING

INGREDIENTS:

- 4 oz boneless, skinless chicken breast
- 1 tablespoon olive oil
- Salt and black pepper (to taste)
- 2 cups romaine lettuce, chopped
- ½ cup chopped cooked bacon
- ¼ cup crumbled blue cheese
- ¼ avocado, sliced
- 1 tomato, chopped
- 1 hard-boiled egg, sliced

COOKING INSTRUCTIONS:

1. Cook the Chicken: Preheat grill pan or skillet over medium-high heat. Season chicken breast with olive oil, salt, and pepper. Grill for 5-6 minutes per side, or until cooked through.
2. Assemble the Salad: On a plate, arrange chopped romaine lettuce. Top with sliced grilled chicken, chopped cooked bacon, crumbled blue cheese, sliced avocado, chopped tomato, and sliced hard-boiled egg.

NUTRITIONAL INFORMATION: (APPROXIMATE VALUES PER SERVING)

Calories: 450

Potassium: 300mg (depending on ingredients)

Protein: 40 grams

Phosphorus: 350mg

Sodium: 300mg (depending on added salt)

TIPS FOR MODIFICATION:

- Portion Control: Enjoy a single serving of chicken breast and adjust portion sizes of other ingredients to manage protein and carbohydrate intake.
- Ingredient Swaps: Consider using lower-sodium bacon or a reduced-fat cheese option.

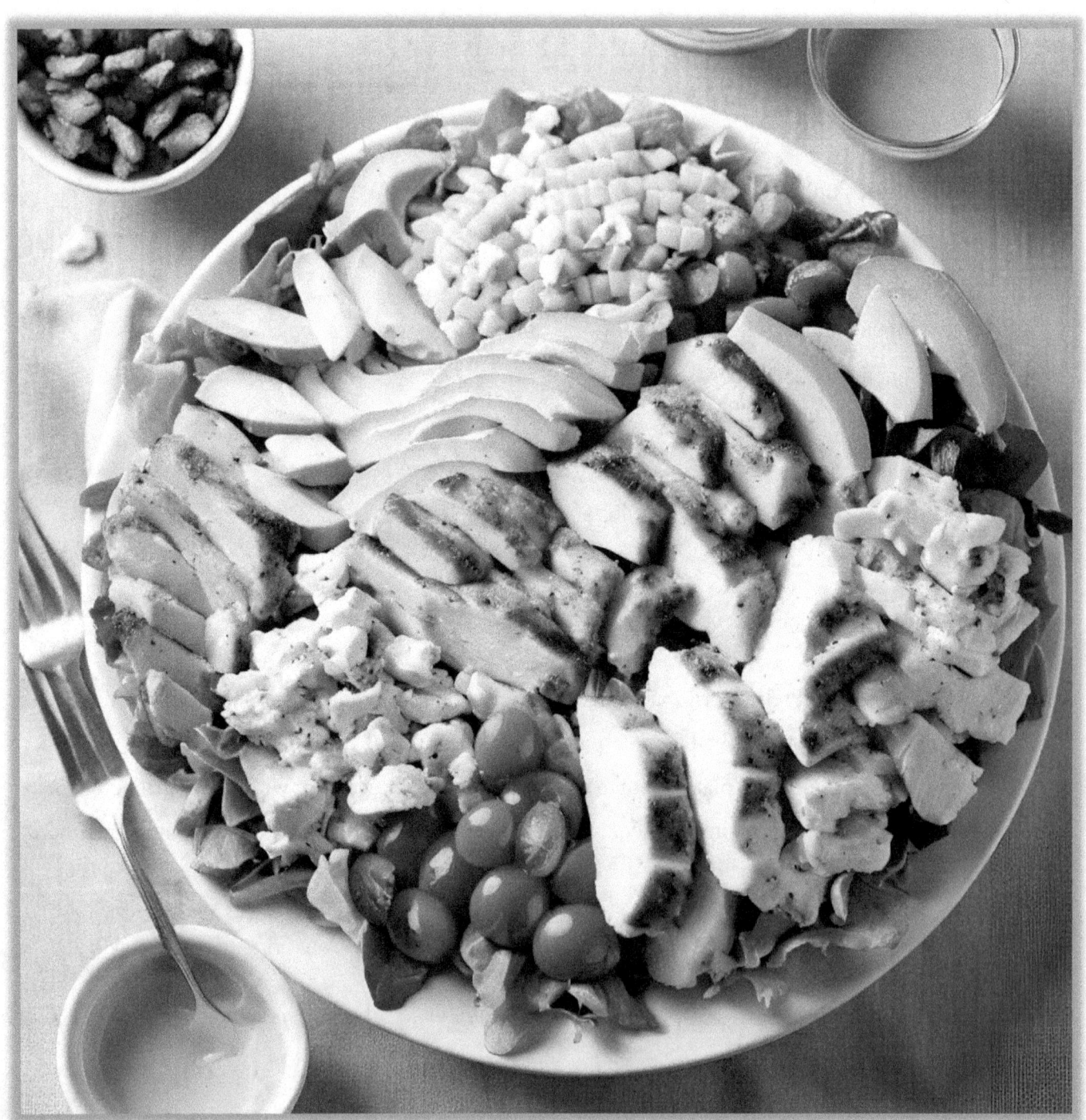

Salmon Salad with Berries and Walnuts

This vibrant salad is perfect for a light and flavorful main course! Packed with protein and healthy fats from salmon, it's bursting with fresh berries and crunchy walnuts. Ideal for those following a CKD diet, this recipe keeps you cool and satisfied.

PREP TIME: 15 MINUTES | COOK TIME: 10-12 MINUTES | YIELDS: 1 SERVING

INGREDIENTS:

- 6 oz salmon fillet (skin-on or skinless)
- 1 tablespoon olive oil
- Salt and black pepper (to taste)
- 1 cup mixed berries (such as raspberries, blueberries, strawberries)
- ¼ cup chopped walnuts
- 2 tablespoons crumbled feta cheese (optional)
- Mixed greens (optional, for a larger salad base)

COOKING INSTRUCTIONS:

1. Cook the Salmon: Preheat oven to 400°F (204°C). Season salmon fillet with olive oil, salt, and pepper. Bake for 10-12 minutes, or until cooked through and flakes easily with a fork.
2. Assemble the Salad: While salmon cooks, arrange mixed greens (if using) on a plate. Top with flaked cooked salmon, fresh berries, and chopped walnuts.
3. Crumble feta cheese over the salad (optional).

NUTRITIONAL INFORMATION: (APPROXIMATE VALUES PER SERVING)

Calories: 400   *Protein: 40 grams*

Potassium: 300mg (depending on ingredients)   *Sodium: 250mg (depending on added salt)*

Phosphorus: 350mg

TIPS FOR MODIFICATION:

- Portion Control: Enjoy a single serving of salmon to manage protein intake.
- Berry Choice: Opt for lower-carbohydrate berries like raspberries or blackberries.

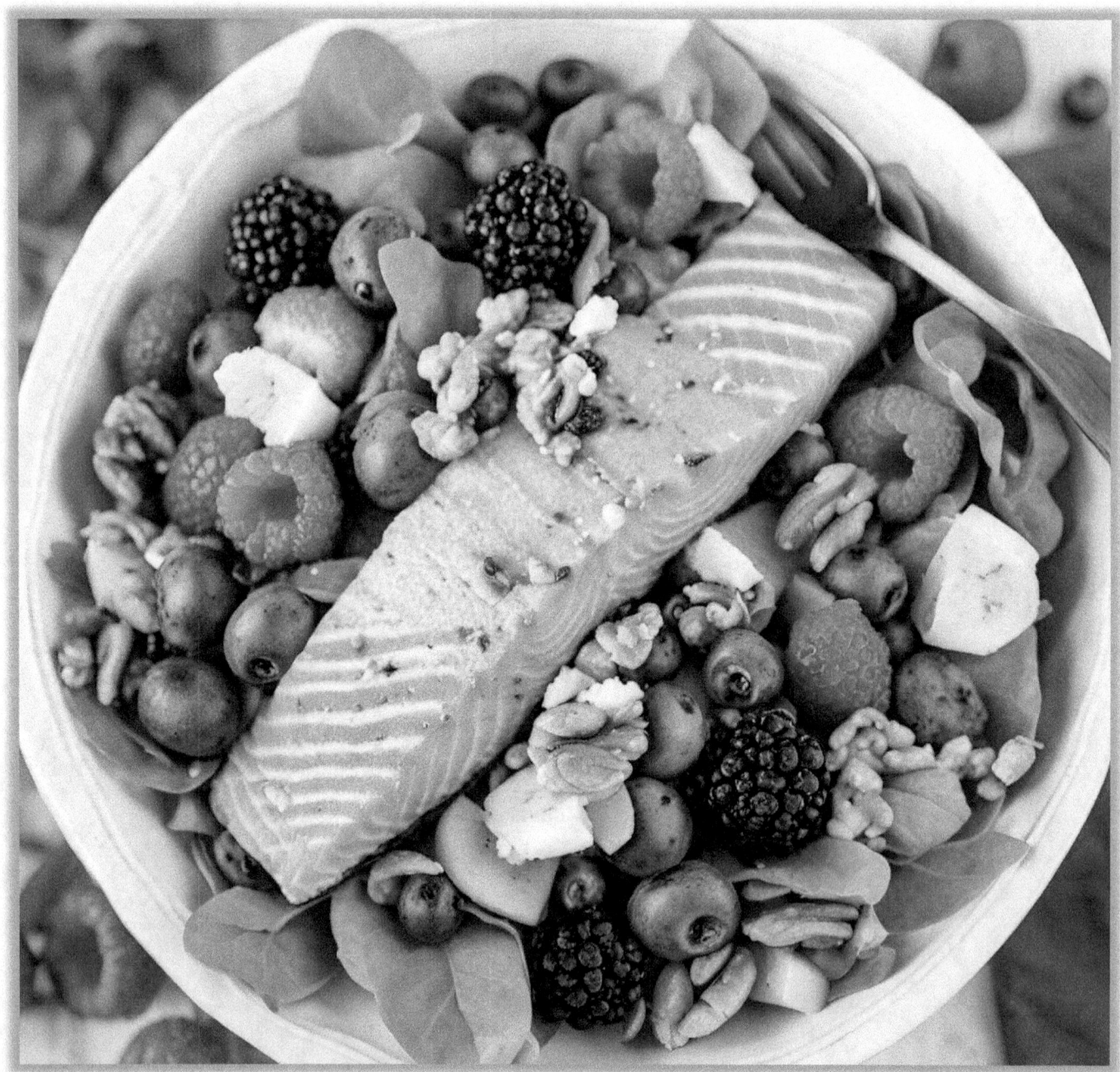

BLT Salad with Turkey Bacon

Enjoy a delicious deconstruction of the BLT in a refreshing salad! This recipe is perfect for a CKD-friendly main course, featuring protein-packed turkey bacon, crisp romaine lettuce, and all the classic BLT fixings.

PREP TIME: 10 MINUTES | COOK TIME: NO COOK TIME (OPTIONAL) | YIELDS: 1 SERVING

INGREDIENTS:

- 4 slices turkey bacon, cooked and chopped
- 2 cups chopped romaine lettuce
- 1 tomato, chopped
- ½ avocado, sliced
- 1 tablespoon mayonnaise (or low-fat option)
- 1 tablespoon lemon juice
- Salt and black pepper (to taste)

Optional Add-Ins:

- Chopped red onion
- Fresh herbs (parsley, dill)
- Crumbled blue cheese (for a stronger flavor)

COOKING INSTRUCTIONS:

1. In a large bowl, combine chopped romaine lettuce, tomato, and avocado.
2. In a separate pan (optional), cook turkey bacon slices until crisp (or use pre-cooked bacon). Crumble the cooked bacon and add it to the salad.
3. In a small bowl, whisk together mayonnaise, lemon juice, salt, and pepper for a light dressing.
4. Pour the dressing over the salad and toss to coat.
5. Enjoy immediately!

NUTRITIONAL INFORMATION: (APPROXIMATE VALUES PER SERVING)

Calories: 350

Phosphorus: 200mg

Protein: 30 grams

Sodium: 150mg (depending on added salt)

Potassium: 300mg (depending on ingredients)

TIPS FOR MODIFICATION:

- Mayonnaise Choice: Opt for a low-fat or light mayonnaise to reduce fat content.
- Portion Control: Enjoy a single serving of turkey bacon and adjust portion sizes of other ingredients to manage protein and carbohydrate intake.

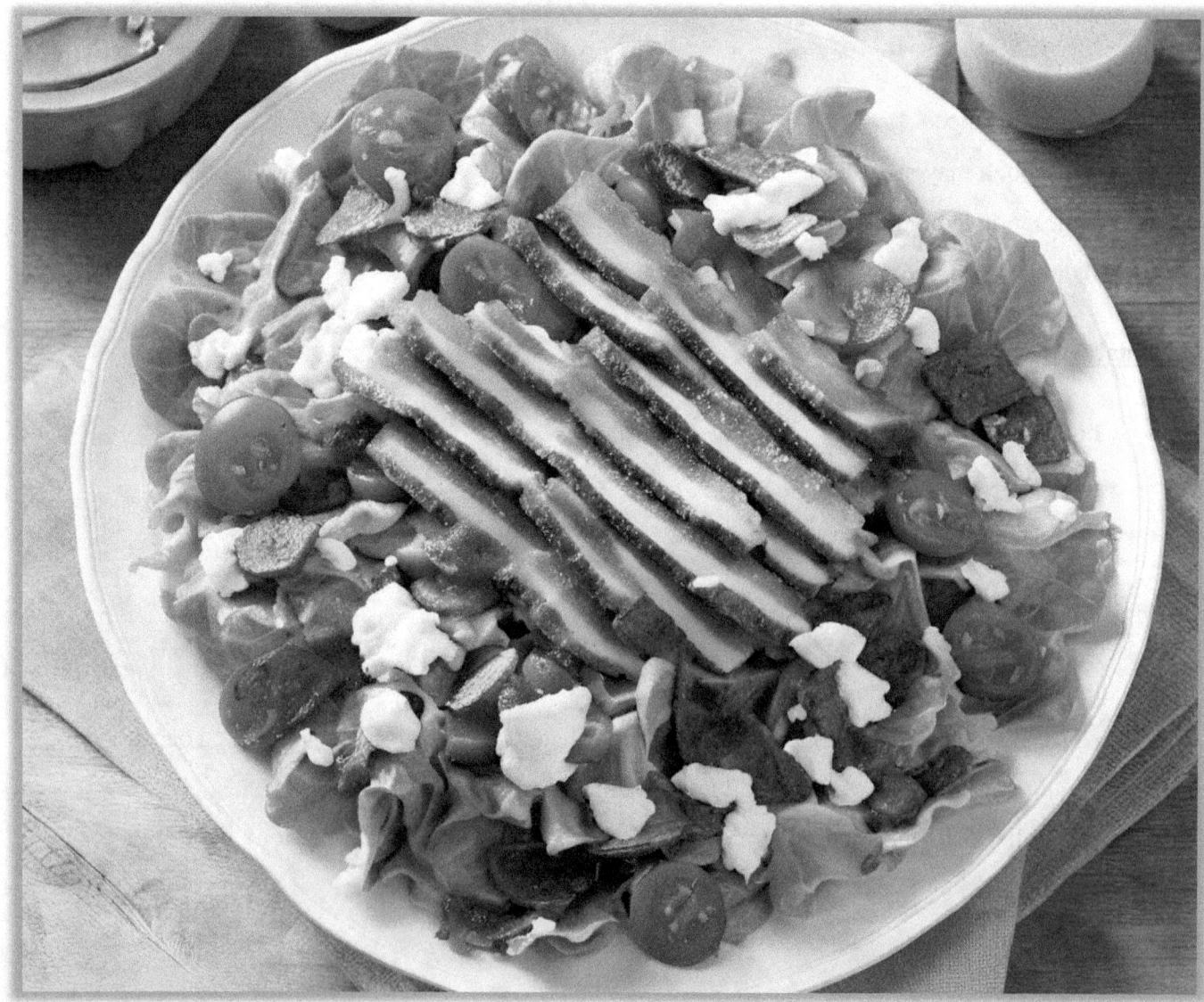

DESSERT

Who says you can't have your cake and eat it too? When it comes to managing Stage 3 kidney disease, enjoying a sweet treat might seem like a distant dream, but fear not! Our dessert recipes are here to prove otherwise.

What to Expect

1. **Fresh and Fruity Delights:** Indulge in the natural sweetness of Fresh Fruit with Vanilla Syrup and the refreshing Watermelon-Blueberry Sorbet. These options are perfect for a light and refreshing end to your meal.
2. **Rich and Decadent Treats:** Satisfy your sweet tooth with richer options like Macadamia Nut Fudge and Chocolate Avocado Pudding. They offer a decadent experience without compromising your dietary needs.
3. **Creamy and Smooth Concoctions:** Dive into the creamy goodness of the Creamy Keto Smoothie and Lemon Ricotta Fluff with Berries. These desserts are smooth, satisfying, and sure to become favorites.
4. **Nutritious and Satisfying:** Enjoy nutritious yet indulgent treats like Sugar-Free Chia Seed Pudding and Spiced Keto Cheesecake Bites. These desserts provide a perfect balance of taste and health benefits.
5. **Quick and Easy:** Some desserts, like Raspberry Fool, are quick and simple to prepare, making them perfect for those moments when you need a fast, delicious treat.

As you explore these kidney-friendly dessert recipes, remember that taking care of your health doesn't mean giving up on enjoyment. With these sweet delights, you can have a treat that's both delicious and good for you. So, get ready to indulge in these guilt-free desserts and add a sweet note to your journey toward better kidney health!

Fresh Fruit with Vanilla Syrup

This recipe features sliced fruit with a touch of vanilla syrup for a satisfying and kidney-friendly treat. Perfect for a light dessert or afternoon pick-me-up!

PREP TIME: 5 MINUTES | COOK TIME: NO COOK TIME | YIELDS: 1 SERVING

INGREDIENTS:

- 1 cup sliced fruits (berries like blueberries or raspberries recommended)
- 1 tablespoon sugar-free vanilla syrup
- Optional: Fresh mint leaves for garnish

COOKING INSTRUCTIONS:

1. In a bowl, combine 1 cup of your chosen sliced fruits. Blueberries and raspberries are good options due to lower potassium content.
2. Drizzle 1 tablespoon of sugar-free vanilla syrup over the fruit slices.
3. Toss gently to coat the fruit evenly.
4. Garnish with a sprig of fresh mint (optional) and enjoy!

NUTRITIONAL INFORMATION: (APPROXIMATE VALUES PER SERVING)

Calories: 80 (depending on fruit and syrup)

Phosphorus: 20mg

Protein: 1 gram

Sodium: 10mg (depending on syrup)

Potassium: 100mg (depending on fruit)

TIPS FOR MODIFICATION:

- Berry Choice: Choose berries lower in potassium like blueberries or raspberries instead of bananas or mangoes.
- Sugar-Free Syrup: opt for sugar-free vanilla syrup to control sugar and carbohydrate intake.

Macadamia Nut Fudge

Indulge in a delightful and healthy dessert with this Macadamia Nut Freezer Fudge recipe! This no-cook treat is packed with heart-healthy fats and satisfying sweetness, making it a perfect choice for a CKD-friendly dessert.

PREP TIME: 5 MINUTES | COOK TIME: NO COOK TIME (NEEDS FREEZING) | YIELDS: 1 SERVING

INGREDIENTS:

- 2 tablespoons unsalted macadamia nuts
- 2 tablespoons unsweetened cocoa powder
- 1 tablespoon heavy cream
- 1 tablespoon sugar-free sweetener (optional, to taste)
- 1 tablespoon water
- Pinch of salt

COOKING INSTRUCTIONS:

1. In a small food processor or blender, grind the macadamia nuts into a fine crumb.
2. In a separate bowl, combine the cocoa powder, heavy cream, water, and salt. Stir until smooth.
3. Add the ground macadamia nuts to the chocolate mixture and fold in gently until well combined.
4. Taste the mixture and add sugar-free sweetener (if using) to achieve your desired level of sweetness.
5. Pour the fudge mixture into a small mold or container lined with parchment paper.
6. Freeze for at least 2 hours, or until solid.

NUTRITIONAL INFORMATION: (APPROXIMATE VALUES PER SERVING)

Calories: 200　　　　　　　　　　　　*Potassium: 50mg*

Protein: 2 grams (from macadamia nuts)　　　*Phosphorus: 100mg*

Sodium: 30mg (depending on ingredients)

TIPS FOR MODIFICATION:

- Portion Control: Enjoy this treat in moderation to manage fat intake.
- Sweetener Options: Consider sugar substitutes like stevia or monk fruit to add sweetness without increasing potassium intake.

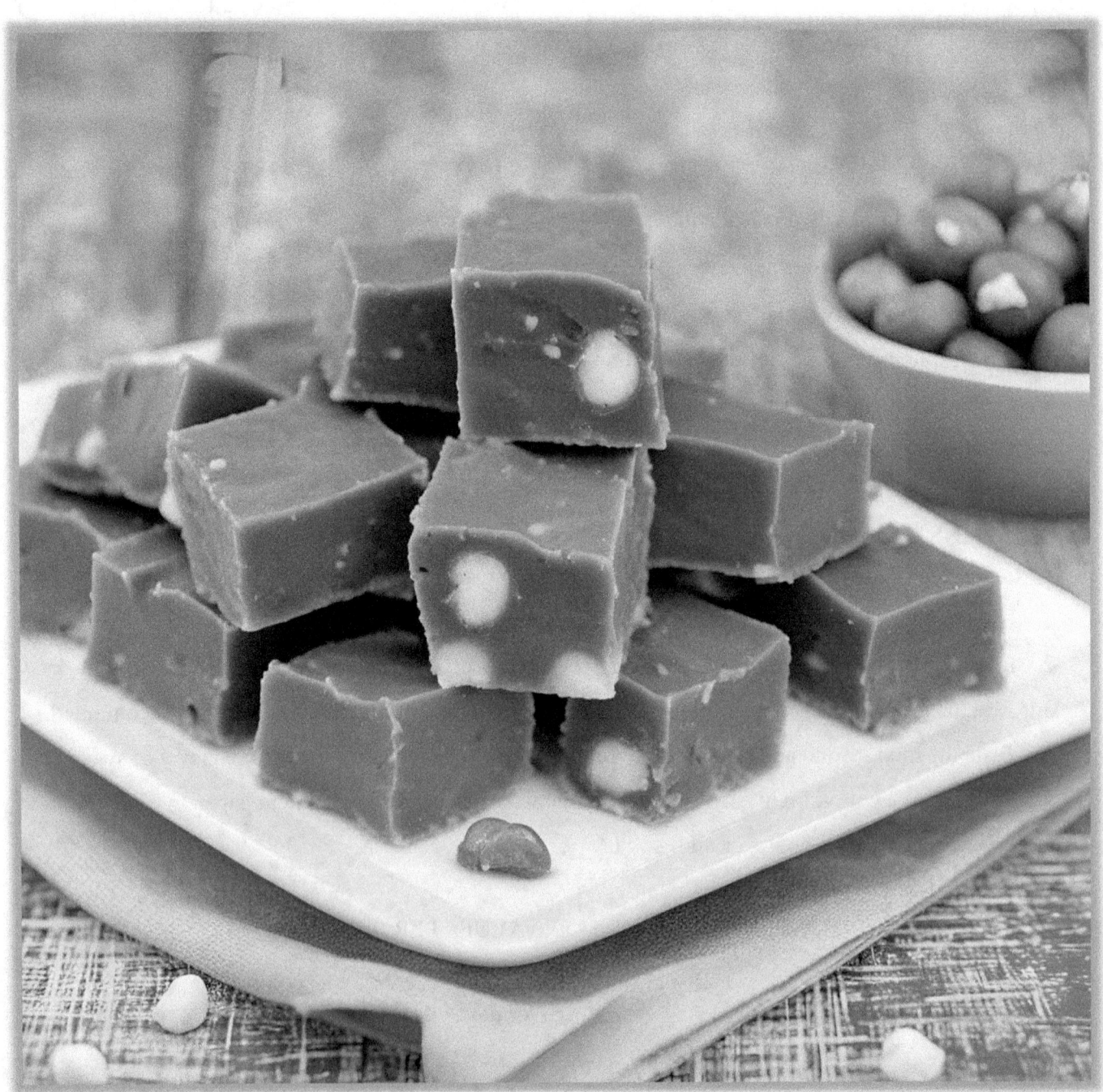

Creamy Keto Smoothie

This Keto Smoothie recipe is packed with healthy fats and protein, making it a perfect way to curb your sweet cravings without compromising your diet.

PREP TIME: 5 MINUTES\COOK TIME: NO COOK TIME | YIELDS: 1 SERVING

INGREDIENTS:

- ½ cup frozen strawberries or raspberries
- ½ cup unsweetened almond milk (or other low-carb milk option)
- ¼ cup plain Greek yogurt (full-fat or low-fat option)
- 1 tablespoon nut butter (almond, peanut, or cashew)
- 1 tablespoon MCT oil (optional)
- Optional: Sugar substitute (to taste)
- Optional: Handful of spinach (for added nutrients)

COOKING INSTRUCTIONS:

1. In a blender, combine ½ cup frozen strawberries or raspberries, ½ cup unsweetened almond milk, ¼ cup plain Greek yogurt, and 1 tablespoon of nut butter.
2. Add MCT oil (optional) for an extra boost of healthy fats.
3. Blend until smooth and creamy.
4. Taste the smoothie and add sugar substitute (if using) to achieve your desired level of sweetness.
5. You can add a handful of spinach for a hidden veggie boost (optional).
6. Pour into a glass and enjoy!

NUTRITIONAL INFORMATION: (APPROXIMATE VALUES PER SERVING)

Calories: 300

Potassium: 150mg (depending on fruit)

Protein: 15 grams (from yogurt and nut butter)

Phosphorus: 200mg

Sodium: 60mg (depending on yogurt)

TIPS FOR MODIFICATION:

- Berry Choice: Choose berries lower in potassium like strawberries or raspberries.
- Milk Choice: Unsweetened almond milk or other low-carb milk options are best.
- Monitor Protein Intake: While Greek yogurt is a good protein source, be mindful of your total protein intake for the day.

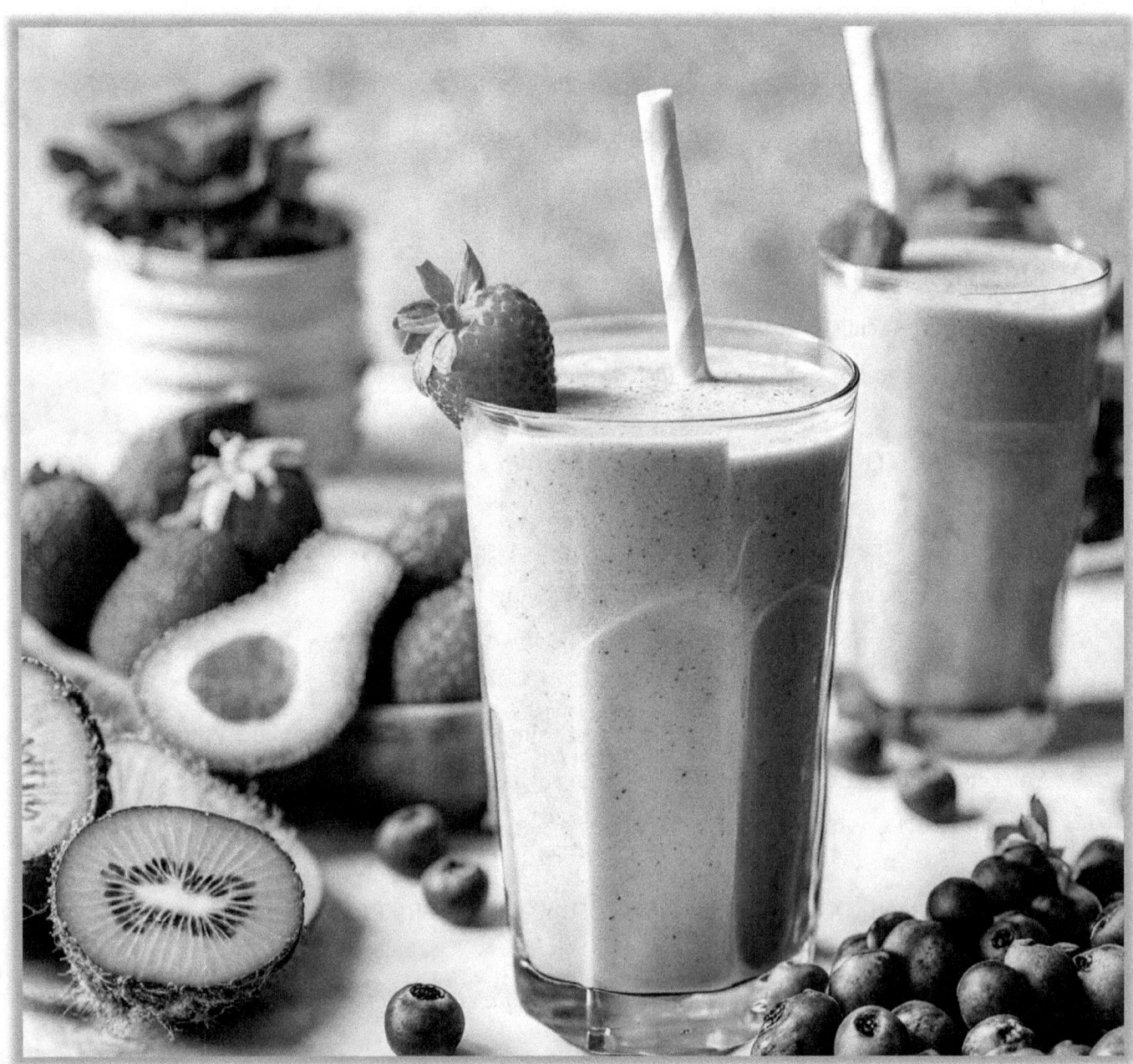

Watermelon-Blueberry Sorbet

Enjoy a cool and flavorful summertime treat with this Watermelon-Blueberry Sorbet recipe! This version is made with a reduced amount of watermelon, making it a more suitable option for a CKD diet.

PREP TIME: 10 MINUTES (FREEZING TIME NOT INCLUDED) | COOK TIME: NO COOK TIME | YIELDS: 1 SERVING

INGREDIENTS:

- 1 cup chopped seedless watermelon
- ½ cup frozen blueberries
- 1 tablespoon lime juice
- Optional: Sugar substitute (to taste)

COOKING INSTRUCTIONS:

1. In a blender, combine 1 cup chopped seedless watermelon, ½ cup frozen blueberries, and 1 tablespoon lime juice.
2. Blend until smooth and scrape down the sides as needed.
3. Taste the mixture and add sugar substitute (if using) to achieve your desired level of sweetness.
4. Pour the sorbet mixture into a shallow container and freeze for at least 4 hours, or until frozen solid.
5. Break up the frozen sorbet with a fork before serving.

NUTRITIONAL INFORMATION: (APPROXIMATE VALUES PER SERVING, ADJUSTED FOR LESS WATERMELON)

Calories: 80

Phosphorus: 20mg

Protein: 1 gram

Sodium: 10mg (depending on ingredients)

Potassium: 100mg (depending on watermelon)

TIPS FOR MODIFICATION:

- Watermelon Portion: This recipe uses less watermelon than traditional sorbet to reduce potassium content.
- Sweetener Options: Consider sugar substitutes like stevia or monk fruit to add sweetness without increasing potassium intake.

Raspberry Fool

Made with lower-potassium ingredients, this creamy treat is a perfect way to end your meal on a sweet note while staying on track with your CKD diet.

PREP TIME: 5 MINUTES | COOK TIME: NO COOK TIME | YIELDS: 1 SERVING

INGREDIENTS:

- ½ cup frozen raspberries
- ¼ cup unsweetened almond milk (or other low-potassium milk option)
- 1 tablespoon heavy whipping cream
- Optional: Sugar substitute (to taste)
- Optional: Fresh mint sprig for garnish

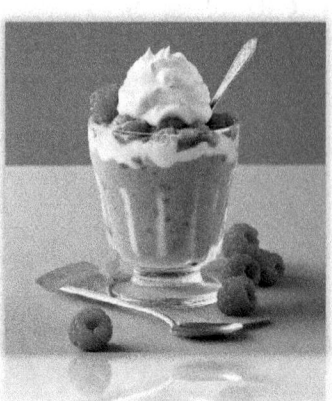

COOKING INSTRUCTIONS:

1. In a blender or food processor, combine ½ cup frozen raspberries and ¼ cup unsweetened almond milk. Blend until smooth.
2. In a separate bowl, whip the heavy whipping cream to soft peaks.
3. Gently fold the whipped cream into the raspberry puree until just combined. Be careful not to overmix.
4. Taste the mixture and add sugar substitute (if using) to achieve your desired level of sweetness.
5. Spoon the Raspberry Fool into a serving dish and garnish with a fresh mint sprig (optional).

NUTRITIONAL INFORMATION: (APPROXIMATE VALUES PER SERVING)

Calories: 120

Phosphorus: 80mg

Protein: 1 gram (from whipping cream)

Sodium: 15mg (depending on ingredients)

Potassium: 75mg (depending on fruit)

TIPS for MODIFICATION:

- Berry Choice: Frozen raspberries are generally lower in potassium than some other berries.
- Milk Choice: Unsweetened almond milk is a lower-potassium option compared to cow's milk. You can explore other low-potassium milk options like oat milk or coconut milk.

Spiced Keto Cheesecake Bites

This recipe offers a delightful and satisfying cheesecake experience in a bite-sized, CKD-friendly format.

PREP TIME: 15 MINUTES (INCLUDING CRUST PREP, OPTIONAL) | COOK TIME: 20 MINUTES | YIELDS: 4-6 SERVINGS

INGREDIENTS:

- For the Crust (Optional):
- 2 tablespoons almond flour
- 1 tablespoon melted unsalted butter
- Pinch of ground cinnamon

For the Cheesecake Filling:

- ¼ cup softened cream cheese (full-fat)
- 1 tablespoon unsweetened almond milk
- 1 tablespoon sugar substitute (powdered)
- ½ teaspoon vanilla extract
- Pinch of ground cinnamon
- Pinch of ground nutmeg

COOKING INSTRUCTIONS:

1. For the Crust (Optional): Combine almond flour, melted butter, and cinnamon in a small bowl. Press the mixture evenly into the bottom of a small baking dish or ramekins. Bake at 350°F (175°C) for 5-7 minutes, or until lightly golden brown. Let cool completely.
2. For the Cheesecake Filling: In a mixing bowl, beat together softened cream cheese, almond milk, sugar substitute, vanilla extract, cinnamon, and nutmeg until smooth and creamy.
3. If using the crust, spoon the cheesecake filling over the cooled crust. If not using a crust, simply portion the filling into small ramekins or molds.
4. Bake at 350°F (175°C) for 15-20 minutes, or until the edges are set and the center is slightly loose.

5. Let cool completely at room temperature, then refrigerate for at least 2 hours or overnight for best results.

NUTRITIONAL INFORMATION: (APPROXIMATE VALUES PER SERVING)

Calories: 150-180 (depending on crust)

Phosphorus: 150mg

Protein: 4 grams (from cream cheese)

Sodium: 60mg (depending on butter)

Potassium: 50mg (depending on almond flour)

TIPS FOR MODIFICATION:

- This recipe uses a small amount of cream cheese and almond milk, keeping portion control in mind.
- Consider sugar substitutes like stevia or monk fruit for sweetness without added potassium.

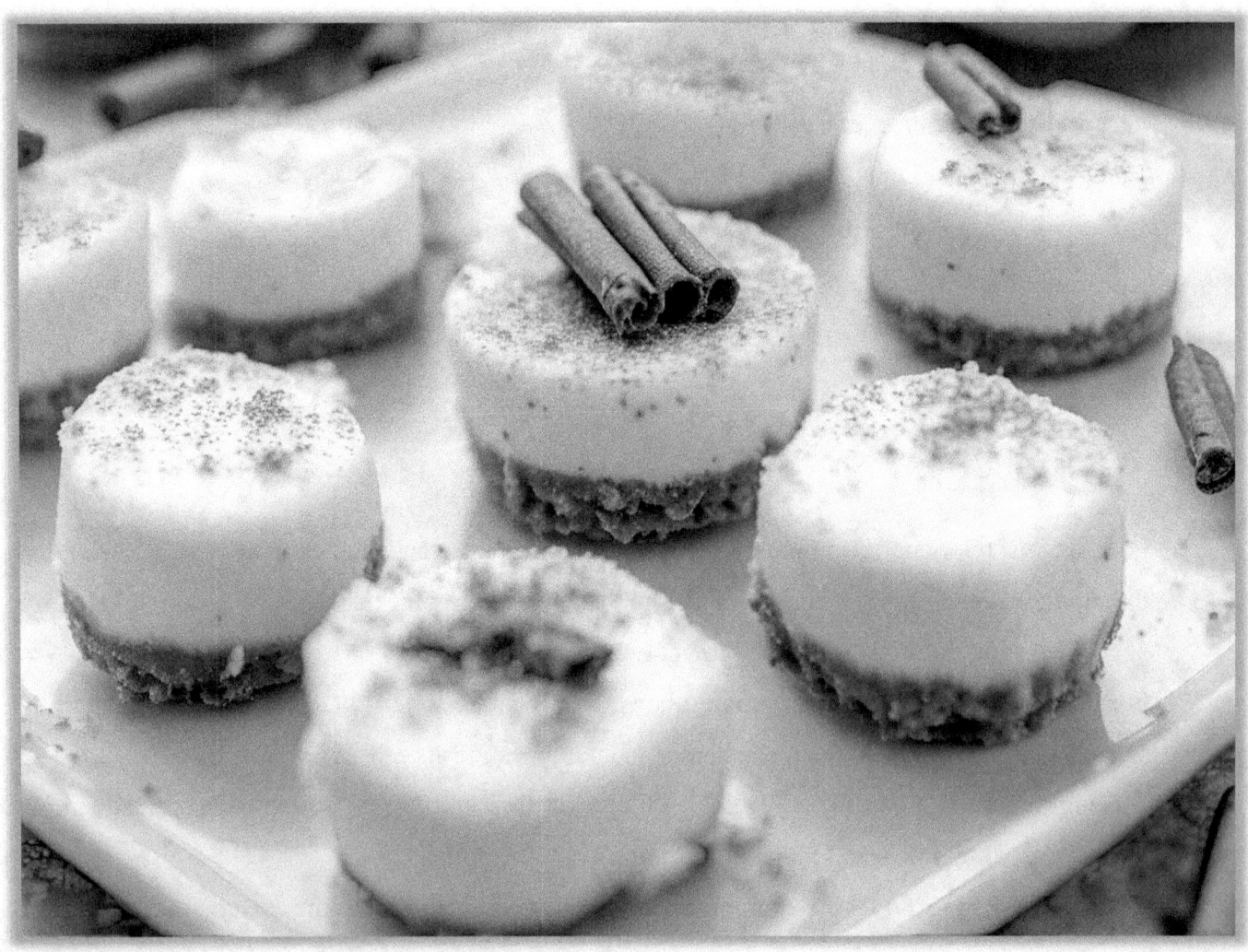

Chocolate Avocado Pudding

This recipe offers a rich and creamy chocolate pudding experience with healthy fats from avocado.

PREP TIME: 5 MINUTES | COOK TIME: NO COOK TIME | YIELDS: 1 SERVING

INGREDIENTS:

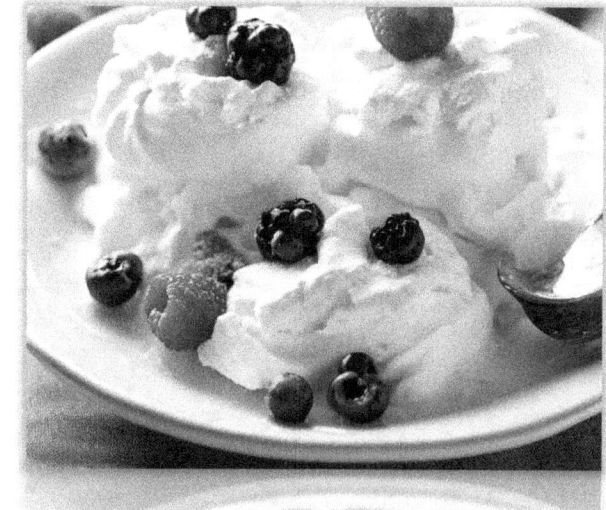

- ½ ripe avocado
- 1-2 tablespoons unsweetened cocoa powder
- 1 tablespoon unsweetened almond milk
- 1 tablespoon sugar substitute (optional)
- ½ teaspoon vanilla extract
- Pinch of salt

COOKING INSTRUCTIONS:

1. In a blender or food processor, combine ½ of a ripe avocado, unsweetened cocoa powder, unsweetened almond milk, sugar substitute (if using), vanilla extract, and salt.
2. Blend until smooth and creamy.
3. Taste and adjust sweetness or cocoa powder content as desired.
4. Pour into a serving dish and enjoy immediately.

NUTRITIONAL INFORMATION: (APPROXIMATE VALUES PER SERVING)

Calories: 200

Phosphorus: 80mg

Protein: 2 grams (from avocado)

Sodium: 30mg (depending on ingredients)

Potassium: 150mg (from avocado)

TIPS FOR MODIFICATION:

- Avocado offers healthy fats while limiting potassium intake compared to some fruits.
- Unsweetened cocoa powder provides a rich chocolate flavor without added sugar.

Lemon Ricotta Fluff with Berries

This recipe is a light and refreshing dessert option with a good protein content from ricotta cheese.

PREP TIME: 5 MINUTES | COOK TIME: NO COOK TIME | YIELDS: 1 SERVING

INGREDIENTS:

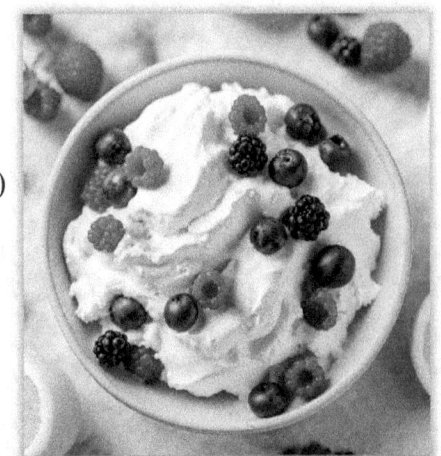

- ¼ cup whole milk ricotta cheese
- 1 tablespoon lemon juice (freshly squeezed or no-sugar-added)
- 1 tablespoon unsweetened almond milk (optional)
- Optional: Sugar substitute (to taste)
- ¼ cup fresh berries (blueberries, raspberries recommended)

COOKING INSTRUCTIONS:

1. In a bowl, combine ricotta cheese, lemon juice, and unsweetened almond milk (if using).
2. Using a whisk or fork, beat the mixture until light and fluffy.
3. Taste and add sugar substitute (if using) to achieve your desired level of sweetness.
4. Spoon the ricotta fluff into a serving dish and top with fresh berries.

NUTRITIONAL INFORMATION: (APPROXIMATE VALUES PER SERVING)

Calories: 180

Phosphorus: 200mg

Protein: 8 grams (from ricotta cheese)

Sodium: 30mg (depending on ricotta cheese)

Potassium: 50mg (depending on berries)

TIPS FOR MODIFICATION:

- Ricotta cheese offers a good source of protein for a satisfying dessert.
- Choose berries lower in potassium like blueberries or raspberries.

Sugar-Free Chia Seed Pudding

Packed with protein and fiber, this pudding is a perfect way to curb your sweet tooth without compromising your CKD diet.

PREP TIME: 5 MINUTES | COOK TIME: NO COOK TIME (NEEDS CHILLING) | YIELDS: 1 SERVING

INGREDIENTS:

- ¼ cup chia seeds
- ½ cup unsweetened almond milk (or other low-potassium milk option)
- 2-3 tablespoons water (depending on desired thickness)
- 1 teaspoon sugar-free sweetener (optional, to taste)
- ½ teaspoon vanilla extract
- Optional: Berries for topping

COOKING INSTRUCTIONS:

1. In a small bowl or jar, combine ¼ cup chia seeds, ½ cup unsweetened almond milk, and 2-3 tablespoons of water (depending on desired thickness).
2. Stir in the sugar-free sweetener (if using) and vanilla extract.
3. Cover the bowl or jar and refrigerate for at least 2 hours, or overnight for a thicker pudding.
4. Once chilled, stir the pudding again and adjust the consistency by adding more water if needed.
5. Top with fresh berries (optional) and enjoy!

NUTRITIONAL INFORMATION: (APPROXIMATE VALUES PER SERVING)

Calories: 150

Phosphorus: 100mg

Protein: 4 grams (from chia seeds)

Sodium: 30mg (depending on milk option)

Potassium: 50mg (depending on milk option)

TIPS FOR MODIFICATION:

- Milk Choice: Unsweetened almond milk is generally lower in potassium than cow's milk. You can explore other low-potassium milk options like oat milk or coconut milk.
- Sweetener Options: Consider sugar substitutes like stevia or monk fruit to add sweetness without increasing potassium intake.

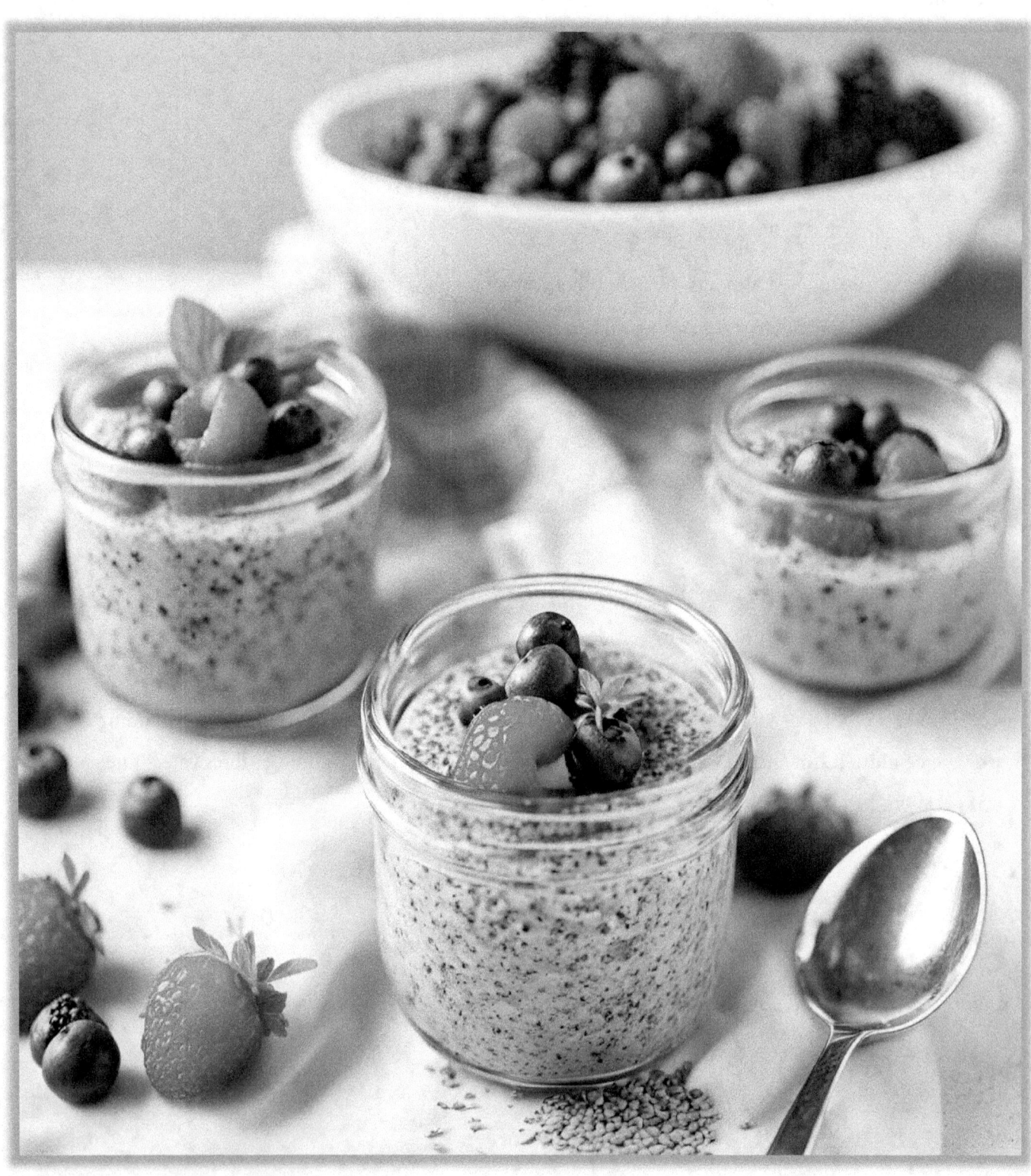

MEAL PLANS AND SHOPPING GUIDES

DAY	BREAKFAST	LUNCH	DINNER	SNACK
WEEK 1				
MON	Apple and Cinnamon Oatmeal	Vegetable Masala	Mexican Street Corn Salad (Esquites)	Curd and Crunch Cottage Cheese
TUE	Berry Oatmeal with Almond Milk	Gumbo Z'Herbes	Veggie Fajitas	Carrot and Creamy Hummus
WED	Scrambled Eggs with Bell Peppers and Mushrooms	Thai Pineapple Salad with Carrot Cashew Dressing	Portobello Steaks with Mashed Cauliflower and Balsamic Arugula	Sweet Yogurt Parfait
THUR	Creamy Breakfast Polenta with Stewed Blackberries	Lemon-Herb Vinaigrette with mixed greens	Italian Pesto Zucchini Noodles	Veggie Straw
FRI	Huevo Ranchero (CKD-Friendly Omelet)	Pumpkin Soup with "Chorizo" Mushrooms and Corn	Pineapple and Veggie Kebabs	Creamy Cottage Cheese & Berry Delight
SAT	Shakshuka	Curry-Ginger Vinaigrette with mixed greens	Refreshing Vinegar Slaw	Rice Cake Remix

SUN	Pecan and Fruit Bowls	Beet Salad with Candied Pecans	Louisiana Remoulade with mixed vegetables	Air-Popped Popcorn Perfection
WEEK 2				
MON	Green Pineapple Smoothie	Smoky Corn and Chile Soup with CKD-Friendly Collard Greens	No-Sodium Umami Sauce with mixed vegetables	Mini Veggie Skewers
TUE	Cottage Cheese with Pineapple and Papaya	Tostada Salad	Summery Pepper Salad	Edamame Energy
WED	High-Fiber Cereal with Berries	Smoky Collard Greens	Main Dish Salad	Almonds and Apple
THUR	Baked Sweet Potato with Chia Seeds	Vegetable Masala	Ginger-Garlic Ramen Bowls	Berry Blast Smoothie
FRI	Pear and Ricotta Toast	Gumbo Z'Herbes	Tortilla-Less Soup	Feta and Dill Cucumber Refreshers
SAT	Low-Sodium Breakfast Burrito	Thai Pineapple Salad with Carrot Cashew Dressing	Smoky Caesar with Charred Romaine	Curd and Crunch Cottage Cheese
SUN	Protein-Free Pancakes	Lemon-Herb Vinaigrette with mixed greens	Jackfruit "Carnitas" Tacos	Carrot and Creamy Hummus
WEEK 3				

MON	Poached Pears with Ginger	Pumpkin Soup with "Chorizo" Mushrooms and Corn	Watermelon Gazpacho	Sweet Yogurt Parfait
TUE	Apple and Cinnamon Oatmeal	Curry-Ginger Vinaigrette with mixed greens	Mushroom Bourguignon	Veggie Straw
WED	Berry Oatmeal with Almond Milk	Beet Salad with Candied Pecans	One-Pan Lemon Garlic Chicken with Veggies	Creamy Cottage Cheese & Berry Delight
THUR	Eggs with Bell Peppers and Mushrooms	Smoky Corn and Chile Soup with CKD-Friendly Collard Greens	Italian Pesto Zucchini Noodles	Rice Cake Remix
FRI	Creamy Breakfast Polenta with Stewed Blackberries	Tostada Salad	Pineapple and Veggie Kebabs	Air-Popped Popcorn Perfection
SAT	Huevo Ranchero (CKD-Friendly Omelet)	Smoky Collard Greens	Refreshing Vinegar Slaw	Mini Veggie Skewers
SUN	Shakshuka	Vegetable Masala	Portobello Steaks with Mashed Cauliflower and Balsamic Arugula	Edamame Energy
	WEEK 4			
MON	Pecan and Fruit Bowls	Gumbo Z'Herbes	Main Dish Salad	Almonds and Apple

TUE	Green Pineapple Smoothie	Thai Pineapple Salad with Carrot Cashew Dressing	Ginger-Garlic Ramen Bowls	Berry Blast Smoothie
WED	Cottage Cheese with Pineapple and Papaya	Lemon-Herb Vinaigrette with mixed greens	Tortilla-Less Soup	Feta and Dill Cucumber Refreshers
THUR	High-Fiber Cereal with Berries	Pumpkin Soup with "Chorizo" Mushrooms and Corn	Smoky Caesar with Charred Romaine	Curd and Crunch Cottage Cheese
FRI	Baked Sweet Potato with Chia Seeds	Curry-Ginger Vinaigrette with mixed greens	Jackfruit "Carnitas" Tacos	Carrot and Creamy Hummus
SAT	Pear and Ricotta Toast	Beet Salad with Candied Pecans	Watermelon Gazpacho	Sweet Yogurt Parfait
SUN	Low-Sodium Breakfast Burrito	Smoky Corn and Chile Soup with CKD-Friendly Collard Greens	Mushroom Bourguignon	Veggie Straw
MON	Protein-Free Pancakes	Tostada Salad	One-Pan Lemon Garlic Chicken with Veggies	Creamy Cottage Cheese & Berry Delight
TUE	Poached Pears with Ginger	Thai Pineapple Salad with Carrot Cashew Dressing	Portobello Steaks with Mashed Cauliflower and Balsamic Arugula	Rice Cake Remix

Congratulations on making it through the month with delicious, kidney-friendly meals!

GROCERY SHOPPING LIST

1. FRUITS	Apples	
	Berries	
	Pineapple	
	Papaya	
	Pears	
	Avocado	
2. VEGETABLES	Bell Peppers	
	Mushrooms	
	Zucchini	
	Carrots	
	Collard Greens	
	Romaine Lettuce	
	Spinach	
	Cauliflower	
	Sweet Potatoes	
3. PROTEINS	Eggs	
	Cottage Cheese	

	Chicken
	Ground Turkey
	Beef
	Cod
	Shrimp
	Tuna
	Tilapia
	Salmon
4. DAIRY AND ALTERNATIVES	Almond Milk
	Ricotta Cheese
	Yogurt
	Feta Cheese
	Cheddar Cheese
5. GRAINS AND CEREALS	Oats
	High-Fiber Cereal
	Rice Cakes
	Bread
	Tortillas

6.	NUTS AND SEEDS	Pecans
		Chia Seeds
		Almonds
7.	SPICES AND CONDIMENTS	Cinnamon
		Ginger
		Lemon
		Dill
8.	SNACKS	Air-Popped Popcorn
		Edamame

With this detailed grocery list, you're all set to embark on a month-long culinary adventure. Happy cooking!

TIPS AND STRATEGIES FOR USING THE GROCERY LIST AND LIFESTYLE CHANGES FOR A KIDNEY DISEASE DIET

Using the Grocery List

1. **Plan Ahead:** Before heading to the grocery store, review the grocery list and meal plan for the week. This ensures you only buy what you need and avoid waste.
2. **Stick to the List:** Avoid impulse buys by sticking strictly to your list. This not only helps you manage your diet more effectively but also saves money.

3. **Shop the Perimeter:** Most fresh produce, dairy, and proteins are found around the perimeter of the store. Focus your shopping here to find the healthiest options.
4. **Read Labels Carefully:** Look for low-sodium, low-potassium, and low-phosphorus options when selecting packaged foods. Avoid items with added sugars and preservatives.
5. **Buy Fresh or Frozen:** Fresh or frozen fruits and vegetables are often healthier choices compared to canned versions, which may contain added sodium or preservatives.
6. **Bulk Buy Wisely:** For items like oats, nuts, and seeds, buying in bulk can be cost-effective. Ensure you have proper storage to keep these items fresh.
7. **Choose Seasonal Produce:** Seasonal fruits and vegetables are often cheaper and more flavorful. Adjust your meal plan slightly if needed to incorporate seasonal produce.
8. **Prep Ahead:** Once you have your groceries, take some time to wash, chop, and store ingredients. This makes meal preparation quicker and more convenient throughout the week.

Lifestyle Changes

1. **Stay Hydrated:** Drink plenty of water throughout the day, but be mindful of your fluid intake if advised by your healthcare provider. Proper hydration helps support kidney function.
2. **Monitor Protein Intake:** While protein is essential, it's important to manage intake to avoid overloading your kidneys. Stick to the protein portions recommended in your recipes.
3. **Limit Sodium:** Excess sodium can increase blood pressure and strain the kidneys. Use herbs and spices to flavor your food instead of salt.
4. **Choose Whole Foods:** Processed foods often contain high levels of sodium, phosphorus, and potassium. Opt for whole, unprocessed foods whenever possible.
5. **Be Mindful of Potassium:** Certain fruits and vegetables are high in potassium, which can be problematic for kidney health. Stick to the recommended foods in your meal plan to manage potassium levels.
6. **Limit Phosphorus:** Phosphorus is found in many dairy products and processed foods. Choose low-phosphorus options and avoid foods with added phosphates.
7. **Maintain a Balanced Diet:** Ensure your diet includes a variety of foods to provide all necessary nutrients. Focus on balance and moderation to support overall health.
8. **Stay Active:** Regular physical activity can improve overall health and support kidney function. Aim for at least 30 minutes of moderate exercise most days of the week.

9. **Follow Medical Advice:** Always follow the guidance of your healthcare provider or dietitian. They can provide personalized advice based on your specific health needs.
10. **Manage Stress:** Chronic stress can negatively impact your health. Incorporate stress-reducing activities such as yoga, meditation, or hobbies you enjoy.

By following these tips and strategies, you can effectively utilize your grocery list and meal plan, while making lifestyle changes that support kidney health. Remember, small, consistent changes can make a significant difference in managing Stage 3 CKD and improving your overall well-being.

APPENDICES

Appendix A: Nutritional Information of Common Ingredients

Understanding the nutritional content of the ingredients you use is essential for managing Stage 3 Chronic Kidney Disease (CKD). This appendix provides a detailed breakdown of the nutritional information of common ingredients found in your meal plans. This will help you make informed choices and better manage your dietary needs.

1. **FRUITS**

Fruits	Serving Size	Calories	Protein (g)	Potassium (mg)	Sodium (mg)	Phosphorus (mg)
Apple	1 medium	95	0.5	195	1	20
Berries	1 cup	85	1.1	114	1.5	18
Pineapple	1 cup	82	0.9	180	2	13
Papaya	1 cup	62	0.7	264	11	14
Pear	1 medium	101	0.6	208	1	20
Avocado	1/2 medium	120	1.5	364	5	36

2. VEGETABLES

Vegetable	Serving Size	Calories	Protein (g)	Potassium (mg)	Sodium (mg)	Phosphorus (mg)
Bell Pepper	1 cup	24	1	210	2	20
Mushrooms	1 cup	15	2.2	223	5	30
Zucchini	1 cup	19	1.5	325	6	33
Carrots	1 cup	52	1.2	390	88	35
Collard Greens	1 cup	63	5.2	220	28	29
Romaine Lettuce	1 cup	8	0.6	116	4	7
Spinach	1 cup	7	0.9	167	24	14
Cauliflower	1 cup	25	2	320	30	44
Sweet Potato	1/2 cup	90	2	475	40	36

3. PROTEINS

Protein Source	Serving Size	Calories	Protein (g)	Potassium (mg)	Sodium (mg)	Phosphorus (mg)
Eggs	1 large	70	6	69	70	95
Cottage Cheese	1/2 cup	110	13	160	400	20
Chicken Breast	3 oz	140	26	210	60	196
Ground Turkey	3 oz	160	22	244	60	200
Beef	3 oz	250	22	240	60	200
Cod	3 oz	70	15	99	60	180
Shrimp	3 oz	80	18	220	119	170
Tuna	3 oz	100	22	300	45	210
Tilapia	3 oz	110	23	378	48	208
Salmon	3 oz	180	19	326	50	220

4. DAIRY AND ALTERNATIVES

Dairy Product	Serving Size	Calories	Protein (g)	Potassium (mg)	Sodium (mg)	Phosphorus (mg)
Almond Milk	1 cup	30	1	180	150	20
Ricotta Cheese	1/2 cup	180	14	187	84	204
Yogurt	1 cup	100	10	380	115	160
Feta Cheese	1 oz	75	4	140	316	96
Cheddar Cheese	1 oz	115	7	28	174	145

5. GRAINS AND CEREALS

Grain	Serving Size	Calories	Protein (g)	Potassium (mg)	Sodium (mg)	Phosphorus (mg)
Oats	1/2 cup	150	5	154	2	180
High-Fiber Cereal	1/2 cup	120	4	140	200	150
Rice Cakes	1 cake	35	0.7	15	0	30

Bread	1 slice	2	4	40	135	50
Tortillas	1 tortilla	3	7	40	190	60

6. NUTS AND SEEDS

Nut/Seed	Serving Size	Calories	Protein (g)	Potassium (mg)	Sodium (mg)	Phosphorus (mg)
Pecans	1 oz	200	3	116	0	70
Chia Seeds	1 tbsp	58	2	44	1	95
Almonds	1 oz	160	6	200	0	136

7. SPICES AND CONDIMENTS

Spice/Condiment	Serving Size	Calories	Protein (g)	Potassium (mg)	Sodium (mg)	Phosphorus (mg)
Cinnamon	1 tsp	6	0.1	11	0	1
Ginger	1 tsp	2	0.1	8	0	1
Lemon	1 medium	17	0.6	80	1	12
Dill	1 tbsp	4	0.2	52	3	2

8. SNACKS

Snack	Serving Size	Calories	Protein (g)	Potassium (mg)	Sodium (mg)	Phosphorus (mg)
Air-Popped Popcorn	1 cup	30	1	30	1	10
Edamame	1/2 cup	120	11	240	15	100

Appendix B: Conversion Charts

Measurements and Substitutions

In cooking, accurate measurements are crucial for the success of recipes, especially when managing a diet for kidney disease. This appendix provides extensive conversion charts and substitution options to help you navigate your cooking process smoothly. Whether you're converting measurements or finding suitable ingredient substitutions, this section has you covered.

Measurement Conversions

Understanding and utilizing the right measurements is key to consistent cooking results. Here are some common conversions for liquid and dry ingredients.

Liquid Measurements

US Standard	Metric Equivalent	Notes
1 teaspoon (tsp)	5 milliliters (ml)	
1 tablespoon (tbsp)	15 milliliters (ml)	3 teaspoons
1 fluid ounce (fl oz)	30 milliliters (ml)	2 tablespoons
1/4 cup	60 milliliters (ml)	
1/3 cup	80 milliliters (ml)	
1/2 cup	120 milliliters (ml)	

2/3 cup	160 milliliters (ml)	
3/4 cup	180 milliliters (ml)	
1 cup	240 milliliters (ml)	
1 pint (pt)	480 milliliters (ml)	2 cups
1 quart (qt)	960 milliliters (ml)	2 pints
1 gallon (gal)	3.8 liters (L)	4 quarts

Dry Measurements

US Standard	Metric Equivalent	Notes
1 ounce (oz)	28 grams (g)	
1 pound (lb.)	454 grams (g)	16 ounces
1 cup (flour)	120 grams (g)	
1 cup (sugar)	200 grams (g)	
1 cup (butter)	227 grams (g)	2 sticks
1 gallon (gal)	3.8 liters (L)	4 quarts

Temperature Conversions

Cooking temperatures are often listed in different units, particularly between Fahrenheit and Celsius. Here's a handy guide for converting temperatures.

Fahrenheit (°F)	Celsius (°C)
200°F	95°C
250°F	120°C
300°F	150°C
350°F	175°C
400°F	200°C
450°F	230°C
500°F	260°C

Ingredient Substitutions

Sometimes you might need to substitute an ingredient due to dietary restrictions, availability, or preference. Below are some common substitutions that can be used without compromising the quality of your dishes.

Dairy Substitutes

If You Have	Use This Instead	Notes
Whole Milk	Almond Milk, Soy Milk, Rice Milk	Use in equal amounts
Heavy Cream	Coconut Cream, Silken Tofu	Blend silken tofu for creamy texture
Butter	Olive Oil, Coconut Oil	Use 3/4 cup oil for every 1 cup butter

Flour Substitutes

If You Have	Use This Instead	Notes
All-Purpose Flour	Whole Wheat Flour, Almond Flour, Oat Flour	Adjust liquid content as needed
Bread Flour	All-Purpose Flour	Slightly different texture, but works in most recipes
Cake Flour	All-Purpose Flour + Cornstarch	For every cup, remove 2 tbsp flour and replace with cornstarch

Egg Substitutes

If You Have	Use This Instead	Notes
1 Egg	1/4 cup Unsweetened Applesauce	Works best in baking
1 Egg	1 tbsp Flaxseed Meal + 3 tbsp Water	Let sit for 5 minutes before using
1 Egg	1/4 cup Mashed Banana	Adds sweetness to recipes

Sugar Substitutes

If You Have	Use This Instead	Notes

White Sugar	Honey, Maple Syrup, Agave Nectar	Use 3/4 cup for every 1 cup sugar, reduce other liquids
Brown Sugar	Coconut Sugar, Muscovado Sugar	Use in equal amounts
Powdered Sugar	Blend White Sugar + Cornstarch	Blend 1 cup sugar with 1 tbsp cornstarch until fine

Sodium Substitutes

Here are some ways to reduce or substitute sodium in your recipes:

If You Have	Use This Instead	Notes
Table Salt	No-Sodium Salt Alternatives, Herbs, and Spices	Experiment with flavor combinations like garlic powder, onion powder, and fresh herbs
Soy Sauce	All-Purpose Flour	Use in reduced quantities and taste as you go
Canned Vegetables	Fresh or Frozen Vegetables	Fresh or frozen are naturally lower in sodium

Summary

This appendix is designed to be your go-to reference for accurate measurements and helpful ingredient substitutions. By utilizing these conversion charts and substitution options, you can ensure that your cooking remains consistent, delicious, and suitable for managing Stage 3 CKD. Remember, precise measurements and smart substitutions can make all the difference in maintaining a healthy diet and enjoying your meals.

CONCLUSION

Congratulations on reaching the end of this kidney-friendly cookbook! Your dedication to managing Stage 3 Chronic Kidney Disease (CKD) through thoughtful and nutritious meals is commendable. The recipes and guidelines provided here are not just about food; they are tools to help you maintain and even improve your kidney health.

The journey of managing kidney health requires vigilance and consistency. Regular check-ups with your healthcare provider are essential to monitor your kidney function and make any necessary adjustments to your diet. Remember, the daily dietary choices you make can have a profound impact on your overall health. By staying committed to a kidney-friendly diet, you can slow the progression of CKD and enhance your quality of life.

Building sustainable, long-term dietary habits is crucial for effectively managing CKD. The recipes in this cookbook are designed to be both satisfying and practical, helping you to form healthy habits that last. Incorporate a wide range of fruits, vegetables, grains, and proteins into your diet to keep it interesting and nutritionally balanced. A diverse diet helps ensure you get all the essential nutrients your body needs. Pay attention to portion sizes to avoid overeating, even with healthy foods. Overeating can lead to weight gain and additional stress on your kidneys. Use the portion guidelines provided in this cookbook to help you stay on track.

Staying properly hydrated is essential for kidney health. Drink the recommended amount of water daily, but avoid excessive fluid intake. Consult your healthcare provider to determine the right amount of fluids for your specific needs. Practice mindful eating by being aware of what and how much you eat. Slow down, savor your meals, and listen to your body's hunger and fullness cues. This can help prevent overeating and improve digestion. Combine healthy eating habits with regular physical activity. Exercise can improve overall health, aid in weight management, and support kidney function. Find activities you enjoy and make them a regular part of your routine.

Staying motivated on your CKD journey can be challenging, but it's crucial for long-term success. Establish realistic, achievable goals for yourself. Whether it's trying a new recipe each week, maintaining your hydration levels, or incorporating more vegetables into your diet, having clear goals can keep you focused and motivated. Keep a food diary or use a nutrition-tracking app to monitor your intake. Tracking your progress can help you stay accountable and make adjustments as needed. Celebrate your successes, no matter how small they may seem.

Knowledge is power. Stay informed about CKD and nutrition by reading articles, joining support groups, and attending workshops or webinars. The more you know, the better equipped you'll be to make informed decisions about your diet and health. Don't be afraid to ask for help. Reach out to family, friends, or support groups for encouragement and assistance. Having a support system can make a significant difference in your journey. Don't be afraid to experiment with new recipes and flavors. Enjoy the process of cooking and discovering new foods that fit your dietary needs. Cooking can be a fun and rewarding experience, and it's a wonderful way to take control of your health.

Maintain a positive mindset. Focus on what you can eat and enjoy rather than what you need to avoid. Approach your diet as a lifestyle change rather than a restriction. Embrace the opportunity to nourish your body with delicious, healthy foods. Your journey with CKD doesn't have to be a struggle. With the right tools, information, and support, you can lead a fulfilling and healthy life. This cookbook is designed to be a companion on your journey, providing you with the recipes, knowledge, and inspiration you need to thrive.

Remember, managing CKD is a marathon, not a sprint. Be patient with yourself, stay committed, and celebrate your progress along the way. Your health and well-being are worth every effort you make. Keep experimenting, keep learning, and keep moving forward. Thank you for choosing this cookbook as your guide. We hope it brings joy to your kitchen and health to your life.

Here's to delicious meals, better health, and a brighter future!